Oliver Sacks

VINTAGE **SACKS**

Oliver Sacks was born in 1933 in London, England, into a family of physicians and scientists, and earned his medical degree at Oxford. Since 1965, he has lived in New York, where he is a practicing neurologist.

In 1966 Dr. Sacks began working in a chronic care facility where he encountered an extraordinary group of patients, many of whom had spent decades in strange, frozen states, like human statues, unable to initiate movement. He recognized these patients as survivors of the great pandemic of sleeping sickness that had swept the world from 1916 to 1927, and treated them with a then-experimental drug, L-DOPA, which enabled them to come back to life. They became the subjects of his book *Awakenings*, which later inspired a play by Harold Pinter and the Oscar-nominated feature film with Robert De Niro and Robin Williams.

Sacks is the author of two collections of case histories from the far borderlands of neurological experience, *The Man Who Mistook His Wife for a Hat* and *An Anthropologist on Mars*, in which he describes patients struggling to live with conditions ranging from Tourette's syndrome to autism, Parkinsonism, musical hallucination, phantom limb syndrome, schizophrenia, and Alzheimer's disease. He has investigated the world of deaf people in *Seeing Voices*, and a rare community of colorblind people in *The Island of the Colorblind*. He has also written about his experiences as a doctor in *Migraine* and as a patient in *A Leg to Stand On*. His most recent books are *Oaxaca Journal* and the autobiographical *Uncle Tungsten: Memories of a Chemical Boyhood*.

His work, which has been supported by the Guggenheim Foundation and the Alfred P. Sloan Foundation, regularly appears in *The New Yorker* and *The New York Review of Books*, as well as various medical journals. *The New York Times* has referred to Dr. Sacks as "the poet laureate of medicine," and in 2002 he was awarded the Lewis Thomas Prize by Rockefeller University, which recognizes the scientist as poet. He is an honorary fellow of both the American Academy of Arts and Letters and the American Academy of Arts and Sciences.

Further information is available
at www.oliversacks.com

*Migraine*

*Awakenings*

*A Leg to Stand On*

*The Man Who Mistook His Wife for a Hat*

*Seeing Voices: A Journey into the World of the Deaf*

*An Anthropologist on Mars*

*The Island of the Colorblind*

*Uncle Tungsten: Memories of a Chemical Boyhood*

*Oaxaca Journal*

# VINTAGE SACKS

Oliver Sacks

VINTAGE BOOKS

A Division of Random House, Inc.

New York

Library of Congress Cataloging-in-Publication Data
Sacks, Oliver W.
Vintage Sacks/Oliver Sacks.
1st Vintage Books ed.
p.   cm.
ISBN 1-4000-3397-7
1. Neurology—Popular works.  2. Neuroscience—Popular works.
RC351.S1953          2004
616.8—dc22
2003057557

*Book design by JoAnne Metsch*

www.vintagebooks.com

Printed in the United States of America
10   9   8   7   6   5   4   3   2   1

# CONTENTS

VINTAGE SACKS

# UNCLE TUNGSTEN

Many of my childhood memories are of metals: these seemed to exert a power on me from the start. They stood out, conspicuous against the heterogeneousness of the world, by their shining, gleaming quality, their silveriness, their smoothness and weight. They seemed cool to the touch, and they rang when they were struck.

I loved the yellowness, the heaviness, of gold. My mother would take the wedding ring from her finger and let me handle it for a while, as she told me of its inviolacy, how it never tarnished. "Feel how heavy it is," she would add. "It's even heavier than lead." I knew what lead was, for I had handled the heavy, soft piping the plumber had left one year. Gold was soft, too, my mother told me, so it was usually combined with another metal to make it harder.

It was the same with copper—people mixed it with tin to produce bronze. Bronze!—the very word was like a trumpet to me, for battle was the brave clash of bronze upon bronze, bronze spears on bronze shields, the great shield of Achilles. Or you could alloy copper with zinc, my mother said, to produce brass. All of us—my mother, my brothers, and I—had our own brass menorahs for Hanukkah. (My father had a silver one.)

I knew copper, the shiny rose color of the great copper cauldron in our kitchen—it was taken down only once a year, when the quinces and crab apples were ripe in the garden and my mother would stew them to make jelly.

I knew zinc: the dull, slightly bluish birdbath in the garden was made of zinc; and tin, from the heavy tinfoil in which sandwiches were wrapped for a picnic. My mother showed me that when tin or zinc was bent it uttered a special "cry." "It's due to deformation of the crystal structure," she said, forgetting that I was five, and could not understand her—and yet her words fascinated me, made me want to know more.

There was an enormous cast-iron lawn roller out in the garden—it weighed five hundred pounds, my father said. We, as children, could hardly budge it, but he was immensely strong and could lift it off the ground. It was always slightly rusty, and this bothered me, for the rust flaked off, leaving little cavities and scabs, and I was afraid the whole roller might corrode and fall apart one day, reduced to a mass of red dust and flakes. I needed to think of metals as stable, like gold—able to stave off the losses and ravages of time.

I would sometimes beg my mother to take out her engagement ring and show me the diamond in it. It flashed like nothing I had ever seen, almost as if it gave out more light than it took in. She would show me how easily it scratched glass, and then tell me to put it to my lips. It was strangely, startlingly cold; metals felt cool to the touch, but the diamond was icy. That was because it conducted heat so well, she said—better than any metal—so it drew the body heat away from one's lips when they touched it. This was a feeling I was never to forget. Another time, she showed me how if one touched a diamond to a cube of ice, it would draw the heat from one's hand into the ice and cut straight through it as if it were butter. My mother told me that diamond was a special form of carbon, like the coal we used in every room in winter. I was puzzled by this—how could black, flaky, opaque coal be the same as the hard, transparent gemstone in her ring?

I loved light, especially the lighting of the shabbas candles on Friday nights, when my mother would murmur a prayer as she lit them. I was not allowed to touch them once they were lit—they were sacred, I was told, their flames were holy, not to be fiddled with. I was mesmerized by the little cone of blue flame at the candle's center—why was it blue? Our house had coal fires, and I would often gaze into the heart of a fire, watching it go from a dim red glow to orange, to yellow, and then I would blow on it with the bellows until it glowed almost white-hot. If it got hot enough, I wondered, would it blaze blue, be blue-hot?

Did the sun and stars burn in the same way? Why did

they never go out? What were they made of? I was reassured when I learned that the core of the earth consisted of a great ball of iron—this sounded solid, something one could depend on. And I was pleased when I was told that we ourselves were made of the very same elements as composed the sun and stars, that some of my atoms might once have been in a distant star. But it frightened me too, made me feel that my atoms were only on loan and might fly apart at any time, fly away like the fine talcum powder I saw in the bathroom.

I badgered my parents constantly with questions. Where did color come from? Why did my mother use the platinum loop that hung above the stove to cause the gas burner to catch fire? What happened to the sugar when one stirred it into the tea? Where did it go? Why did water bubble when it boiled? (I liked to watch water set to boil on the stove, to see it quivering with heat before it burst into bubbles.)

My mother showed me other wonders. She had a necklace of polished yellow pieces of amber, and she showed me how, when she rubbed them, tiny pieces of paper would fly up and stick to them. Or she would put the electrified amber against my ear, and I would hear and feel a tiny snap, a spark.

My two older brothers Marcus and David, nine and ten years older than I, were fond of magnets and enjoyed demonstrating these to me, drawing the magnet beneath a piece of paper on which were strewn powdery iron filings.

I never tired of the remarkable patterns that rayed out from the poles of the magnet. "Those are lines of force," Marcus explained to me—but I was none the wiser.

Then there was the crystal radio my brother Michael gave me, which I played with in bed, jiggling the wire on the crystal until I got a station loud and clear. And the luminous clocks—the house was full of them, because my uncle Abe had been a pioneer in the development of luminous paints. These, too, like my crystal radio, I would take under the bedclothes at night, into my private, secret vault, and they would light up my cavern of sheets with an eerie, greenish light.

All these things—the rubbed amber, the magnets, the crystal radio, the clock dials with their tireless coruscations—gave me a sense of invisible rays and forces, a sense that beneath the familiar, visible world of colors and appearances there lay a dark, hidden world of mysterious laws and phenomena.

Whenever we had "a fuse," my father would climb up to the porcelain fusebox high on the kitchen wall, identify the fused fuse, now reduced to a melted blob, and replace it with a new fuse of an odd, soft wire. It was difficult to imagine that a metal could melt—could a fuse really be made from the same material as a lawn roller or a tin can?

The fuses were made of a special alloy, my father told me, a combination of tin and lead and other metals. All of these had relatively low melting points, but the melting point of their alloy was lower still. How could this be so, I wondered? What was the secret of this new metal's strangely low melting point?

For that matter, what was electricity, and how did it flow? Was it a sort of fluid like heat, which could also be conducted? Why did it flow through the metal but not the porcelain? This, too, called for explanation.

My questions were endless, and touched on everything, though they tended to circle around, again and again, to my obsession, the metals. Why were they shiny? Why smooth? Why cool? Why hard? Why heavy? Why did they bend, not break? Why did they ring? Why could two soft metals like zinc and copper, or tin and copper, combine to produce a harder metal? What gave gold its goldness, and why did it never tarnish? My mother was patient, for the most part, and tried to explain, but eventually, when I exhausted her patience, she would say, "That's all I can tell you—you'll have to quiz Uncle Dave to learn more."


We had called him Uncle Tungsten for as long as I could remember, because he manufactured lightbulbs with filaments of fine tungsten wire. His firm was called Tungstalite, and I often visited him in the old factory in Farringdon and watched him at work, in a wing collar, with his shirtsleeves rolled up. The heavy, dark tungsten powder would be pressed, hammered, sintered at red heat, then drawn into finer and finer wire for the filaments. Uncle's hands were seamed with the black powder, beyond the power of any washing to get out (he would have to have the whole thickness of epidermis removed, and even this, one suspected, would not have been enough). After thirty years of working with tungsten, I imagined, the heavy element was in his lungs and bones, in every vessel and viscus, every tissue of his body. I thought of this as a wonder, not a curse—his body invigorated and fortified by the mighty element, given a strength and enduringness almost more than human.

Whenever I visited the factory, he would take me around the machines, or have his foreman do so. (The foreman was a short, muscular man, a Popeye with enormous forearms, a palpable testament to the benefits of working with tungsten.) I never tired of the ingenious machines, always beautifully clean and sleek and oiled, or the furnace where the black powder was compacted from a powdery incoherence into dense, hard bars with a grey sheen.

During my visits to the factory, and sometimes at home, Uncle Dave would teach me about metals with little experiments. I knew that mercury, that strange liquid metal, was incredibly heavy and dense. Even lead floated on it, as my uncle showed me by floating a lead bullet in a bowl of quicksilver. But then he pulled out a small grey bar from his pocket, and to my amazement, this sank immediately to the bottom. That, he said, was *his* metal, tungsten.

Uncle loved the density of the tungsten he made, and its refractoriness, its great chemical stability. He loved to handle it—the wire, the powder, but the massy little bars and ingots most of all. He caressed them, balanced them (tenderly, it seemed to me) in his hands. "Feel it, Oliver," he would say, thrusting a bar at me. "Nothing in the world feels like sintered tungsten." He would tap the little bars and they would emit a deep clink. "The sound of tungsten," Uncle Dave would say, "nothing like it." I did not know whether this was true, but I never questioned it.

As the youngest of almost the youngest (I was the last of four, and my mother the sixteenth of eighteen), I was born almost a hundred years after my maternal grandfather and never knew him. He was born Mordechai Fredkin, in 1837, in a small village in Russia. As a youth he managed to avoid being impressed into the Cossack army and fled Russia using the passport of a dead man named Landau; he was just sixteen. As Marcus Landau, he made his way to Paris and then Frankfurt, where he married (his wife was sixteen too). Two years later, in 1855, now with the first of their children, they moved to England.

My mother's father was, by all accounts, a man drawn equally to the spiritual and the physical. He was by profession a boot and shoe manufacturer, a *shochet* (a kosher slaughterer), and later a grocer—but he was also a Hebrew scholar, a mystic, an amateur mathematician, and an inventor. He had a wide-ranging mind: he published a newspaper, the *Jewish Standard,* in his basement, from 1888 to 1891; he was interested in the new science of aeronautics and corresponded with the Wright brothers, who paid him a visit when they came to London in the early 1900s (some of my uncles could still remember this). He had a passion, my aunts and uncles told me, for intricate arithmetical calculations, which he would do in his head while lying in the bath. But he was drawn above all to the invention of lamps—safety lamps for mines, carriage lamps, streetlamps—and he patented many of these in the 1870s.

A polymath and autodidact himself, Grandfather was passionately keen on education—and, most especially, a scientific education—for all his children, for his nine daughters no less than his nine sons. Whether it was this or the sharing of his own passionate enthusiasms, seven of his sons were eventually drawn to mathematics and the physical sciences, as he was. His daughters, by contrast, were by and large drawn to the human sciences—to biology, to medicine, to education and sociology. Two of them founded schools. Two others were teachers. My mother was at first torn between the physical and the human sciences: she was particularly attracted to chemistry as a girl (her older brother Mick had just begun a career as a chemist), but later became an anatomist and surgeon. She never lost her love of, her feelings for, the physical sciences, nor the desire to go beneath the surfaces of things, to explain. Thus the thousand and one questions I asked as a child were seldom met by impatient or peremptory answers, but careful ones which enthralled me (though they were often above my head). I was encouraged from the start to interrogate, to investigate.

Given all my aunts and uncles (and a couple more on my father's side), my cousins numbered almost a hundred; and since the family, for the most part, was centered in London (though there were far-flung American, Continental, and South African branches), we would all meet frequently, tribally, on family occasions. This sense of extended family was one I knew and enjoyed as far back as memory goes, and it went with a sense that it was our business, the family business, to ask questions, to be "scientific," just as we were Jewish or English. I was among the youngest of the cousins—I had cousins in South Africa who were forty-five years my senior—and some of these cousins were already practicing scientists or mathematicians; others, only a little older than myself, were already in love with science. One cousin was a young physics teacher; three were reading chemistry at university; and one, a precocious fifteen-year-old, was showing great mathematical promise. All of us, I could not help imagining, had a bit of the old man in us.

# STINKS AND BANGS

Attracted by the sounds and flashes and smells coming from my lab, David and Marcus, now medical students, sometimes joined me in experiments—the nine- and ten-year age differences between us hardly mattered at these times. On one occasion, as I was experimenting with hydrogen and oxygen, there was a loud explosion, and an almost invisible sheet of flame, which blew off Marcus's eyebrows completely. But Marcus took this in good part, and he and David often suggested other experiments.

We mixed potassium perchlorate with sugar, put it on the back step, and banged it with a hammer. This caused a most satisfying explosion. It was trickier with nitrogen tri-iodide, easily made by adding concentrated ammonia to iodine, catching the nitrogen tri-iodide on filter paper, and drying it with ether. Nitrogen tri-iodide was incredibly touch-sensitive; one had only to touch it with a stick—a *long* stick (or even a feather)—and it would explode with surprising violence.

We made a "volcano" together with ammonium dichro-mate, setting fire to a pyramid of the orange crystals, which then flamed, furiously, becoming red-hot, throwing off showers of sparks in all directions, and swelling porten-tously, like a miniature volcano erupting. Finally, when it had died down, there was, in place of the neat pyramid of crystals, a huge fluffy pile of dark green chromic oxide.

Another experiment, suggested by David, involved pour-ing concentrated, oily sulfuric acid on a little sugar, which instantly turned black, heated, steamed, and expanded, forming a monstrous pillar of carbon rising high above the rim of the beaker. "Beware," David said, as I gazed at this transformation. "*You'll* be turned into a pillar of carbon if you get the acid on yourself." And then he told me horror stories, probably invented, of vitriol throwings in East Lon-don, and patients he had seen coming into the hospital with their entire faces all but burned off. (I was not quite sure whether to believe him, for when I was younger he had told me that if I looked at the Kohanim as they were blessing us in the shul—their heads were covered with a large shawl, a tallis, as they prayed, for they were irradiated, at this moment, by the blinding light of God—my eyes would melt in their sockets and run down my cheeks like fried eggs.)[1]

---

[1] I read John Hersey's *Hiroshima* a few years later, and I was struck by this passage:

> When he had penetrated the bushes, he saw there were about twenty men, and they were all in exactly the same nightmarish state: their faces were wholly burned, their eyesockets were hollow, the fluid from their melted eyes had run down their cheeks. (They must have had their faces upturned when the bomb went off. . . .)

I spent a good deal of my time in the lab examining chemical colors and playing with them. There were certain colors that held a special, mysterious power for me—this was especially so of very deep and pure blues. As a child I had loved the strong, bright blue of the Fehling's solution in my father's dispensary, just as I had loved the cone of pure blue at the center of a candle flame. I found I could produce very intense blues with some cobalt compounds, with cuprammonium compounds, and with complex iron compounds like Prussian blue.

But the most mysterious and beautiful of all the blues for me was that produced by dissolving alkali metals in liquid ammonia (Uncle Dave showed me this). The fact that metals *could* be dissolved at all was startling at first, but the alkali metals were all soluble in liquid ammonia (some to an astounding degree—cesium would completely dissolve in a third its weight of ammonia). When the solutions became more concentrated, they suddenly changed character, turning into lustrous bronze-colored liquids that floated on the blue—and in this state they conducted electricity as well as liquid metal like mercury. The alkaline earth metals would work as well, and it did not matter whether the solute was sodium or potassium, calcium or barium—the ammoniacal solutions, in every case, were an identical deep blue, suggesting the presence of some substance, some structure, something common to them all. It was like the color of the azurite in the Geological Museum, the very color of heaven.

Many of the so-called transition elements infused their compounds with characteristic colors—most cobalt and manganese salts were pink; most copper salts deep blue or greenish blue; most iron salts pale green and nickel salts a deeper green. Similarly, in minute amounts, transition elements gave many gems their particular colors. Sapphires, chemically, were basically nothing but corundum, a colorless aluminum oxide, but they could take on every color in the spectrum—with a little bit of chromium replacing some of the aluminum, they would turn ruby red; with a little titanium, a deep blue; with ferrous iron, green; with ferric iron, yellow. And with a little vanadium, the corundum began to resemble alexandrite, alternating magically between red and green—red in incandescent light, green in daylight. With certain elements, at least, the merest smattering of atoms could produce a characteristic color. No chemist could have "flavored" corundum with such delicacy, a few atoms of this, a few ions of that, to produce an entire spectrum of colors.

There were only a handful of these "coloring" elements—titanium, vanadium, chromium, manganese, iron, cobalt, nickel, and copper, so far as I could see, being the main ones. They were, I could not help noticing, all bunched together in terms of atomic weight—though whether this meant anything, or was just a coincidence, I had no idea at the time. It was characteristic of all of these, I learned, that they had a number of possible valency states, unlike most of the other elements, which had only one. Sodium, for instance, would combine with chlorine in only one way, one atom of sodium to one of chlorine. But there were two combinations of iron and chlorine: an atom of iron could combine with two atoms of chlorine to form ferrous chloride ($FeCl_2$) or with three atoms of chlorine to form ferric chloride ($FeCl_3$). These two chlorides were very different in many ways, including color.

Because it had four strikingly different valencies or oxidation states, and it was easy to transform these into one another, vanadium was an ideal element to experiment with. The simplest way of reducing vanadium was to start with a test tube full of (pentavalent) ammonium vanadate in solution and add small lumps of zinc amalgam. The amalgam would immediately react, and the solution would turn from yellow to royal blue (the color of tetravalent vanadium). One could remove the amalgam at this point, or let it react further, till the solution turned green, the color of trivalent vanadium. If one waited still longer, the green would disappear and be replaced by a beautiful lilac, the color of divalent vanadium. The reverse experiment was even more beautiful, especially if one layered potassium permanganate, a deep purple layer, over the delicate lilac; this would be oxidized over a period of hours and form separate layers, one above the other, of lilac divalent vanadium on the bottom, then green trivalent vanadium, then blue tetravalent vanadium, then yellow pentavalent vanadium (and on top of this, a rich brown layer of the original permanganate, now brown because it was mixed with manganese dioxide).

These experiences with color convinced me that there was a very intimate (if unintelligible) relation between the atomic character of many elements and the color of their compounds or minerals. The same color would show itself whatever compound one looked at. It could be, for example, manganous carbonate, or nitrate, or sulfate, or whatever—all had the identical pink of the divalent manganous ion (the permanganates, by contrast, where the manganese ion was heptavalent, were all deep purple). And from this I got a vague feeling—it was certainly not one that I could formulate with any precision at the time—that the color of these metal ions, their chemical color, was related to the specific state of their atoms as they moved from one oxidation state to another. What was it about the transition elements, in particular, that gave them their characteristic colors? Were these substances, their atoms, in some way "tuned"?[2]

---

[2]Such thoughts about "tuning," I was later to read, had first been raised in the eighteenth century by the mathematician Euler, who had ascribed the color of objects to their having "little particles" on their surface—atoms—tuned to respond to light of different frequencies. Thus an object would look red because its "particles" were tuned to vibrate, resonate, to the red rays in the light that fell on it:

> The nature of the radiation by which we see an opaque object does not depend on the source of light but on the vibratory motion of the very small particles [atoms] of the object's surface. These little particles are like stretched strings, tuned to a certain frequency, which vibrate in response to a similar vibration of the air even if no one plucks them.

A lot of chemistry seemed to be about heat—sometimes a demand for heat, sometimes the production of heat. Often one needed heat to start a reaction, but then it would go by itself, sometimes with a vengeance. If one simply mixed iron filings and sulfur, nothing happened—one could still pull out the iron filings from the mixture with a magnet. But if one started to heat the mixture, it suddenly glowed, became incandescent, and something totally new—iron sulfide—was created. This seemed a basic, almost primordial reaction, and I imagined that it occurred on a vast scale in the earth, where molten iron and sulfur came into contact.

One of my earliest memories (I was only two at the time) was of seeing the Crystal Palace burn. My brothers took me to see it from Parliament Hill, the highest point on Hampstead Heath, and all around the burning palace the night sky was lit up in a wild and beautiful way. And every November 5, in memory of Guy Fawkes, we would

---

Just as the stretched string is excited by the same sound that it emits, the particles of the surface begin to vibrate in tune with the incident radiation and to emit their own waves in every direction.

David Park, in *The Fire Within the Eye: A Historical Essay on the Nature and Meaning of Light,* writes of Euler's theory:

I think this was the first time anyone who believed in atoms ever suggested that they have a vibrating internal structure. The atoms of Newton and Boyle are clusters of hard little balls, Euler's atoms are like musical instruments. His clairvoyant insight was rediscovered much later, and when it was, nobody remembered who had it first.

have fireworks in the garden—little sparklers full of iron dust; Bengal lights in red and green; and bangers, which made me whimper with fear and want to crawl, as our dog would, under the nearest shelter. Whether it was these experiences, or whether it was a primordial love of fire, it was flames and burnings, explosions and colors, which had such a special (and sometimes fearful) attraction for me.

I liked mixing iodine and zinc, or iodine and antimony—no added heat was needed here—and seeing how they heated up spontaneously, sending a cloud of purple iodine vapor above them. The reaction was more violent if one used aluminum rather than zinc or antimony. If I added two or three drops of water to the mixture, it would catch fire and burn with a violet flame, spreading fine brown iodide powder over everything.

Magnesium, like aluminum, was a metal whose paradoxes intrigued me: strong and stable enough in its massive form to be used in airplane and bridge construction, but almost terrifyingly active once oxidation, combustion, got started. One could put magnesium in cold water, and nothing would happen. If one put it in hot water, it would start to bubble hydrogen; but if one lit a length of magnesium ribbon, it would continue to burn with dazzling brilliance *under* the water, or even in normally flame-suffocating carbon dioxide. This reminded me of the incendiary bombs used during the war, and how they could not be quenched by carbon dioxide or water, or even by sand. Indeed, if one heated magnesium with sand, silicon dioxide—and what could be more inert than sand?—the magnesium would burn brilliantly, pulling the oxygen out of the sand, producing elemental silicon or a mixture of silicon with magnesium silicide. (Nonetheless, sand was used to suffocate ordinary fires that had been started by incendiary bombs, even if it was useless against burning magnesium itself, and one saw sand buckets everywhere in London during the war; every house had its own.) If one then tipped the silicide into dilute hydrochloric acid, it would react to form a spontaneously inflammable gas, hydrogen silicide, or silane— bubbles of this would rise through the solution, forming smoke rings, and ignite with little explosions as they reached the surface.

For burning, one used a very long-stemmed "deflagrating" spoon, which one could lower gingerly, with its thimbleful of combustible, into a cylinder of air, or oxygen, or chlorine, or whatever. The flames were all better and brighter if one used oxygen. If one melted sulfur and then lowered it into the oxygen, it took fire and burned with a bright blue flame, producing pungent, titillating, but suffocating sulfur dioxide. Steel wool, purloined from the kitchen, was surprisingly inflammable—this, too, burned brilliantly in oxygen, producing showers of sparks like the sparklers on Guy Fawkes night, and a dirty brown dust of iron oxide.

With chemistry such as this, one was playing with fire, in the literal as well as the metaphorical sense. Huge energies, plutonic forces, were being unleashed, and I had a thrilling but precarious sense of being in control—some-times just. This was especially so with the intensely exother-mic reactions of aluminum and magnesium; they could be used to reduce metallic ores, or even to produce elemental silicon from sand, but a little carelessness, a miscalculation, and one had a bomb on one's hands.

Chemical exploration, chemical discovery, was all the more romantic for its dangers. I felt a certain boyish glee in play-ing with these dangerous substances, and I was struck, in my reading, by the range of accidents that had befallen the pioneers. Few naturalists had been devoured by wild ani-mals or stung to death by noxious plants or insects; few physicists had lost their eyesight gazing at the heavens, or broken a leg on an inclined plane; but many chemists had lost their eyes, limbs, and even their lives, usually through producing inadvertent explosions or toxins. All the early investigators of phosphorus had burned themselves severely. Bunsen, investigating cacodyl cyanide, lost his right eye in an explosion, and very nearly his life. Several later exper-imenters, like Moissan, trying to make diamond from graphite in intensely heated, high-pressure "bombs," threat-ened to blow themselves and their fellow workers to king-dom come. Humphry Davy, one of my particular heroes, had been nearly asphyxiated by nitrous oxide, poisoned himself with nitrogen peroxide, and severely inflamed his lungs with hydrofluoric acid. Davy also experimented with the first "high" explosive, nitrogen trichloride, which had cost many people fingers and eyes. He discovered several new ways of making the combination of nitrogen and chlorine, and caused a violent explosion on one occasion while he was visiting a friend. Davy himself was partially blinded, and did not recover fully for another four months. (We were not told what damage was done to his friend's house.)

*The Discovery of the Elements* devoted an entire section to "The Fluorine Martyrs." Although elemental chlorine had been isolated from hydrochloric acid in the 1770s, its far more active cousin, fluorine, was not so easily obtained. All the early experimenters, I read, "suffered the frightful torture of hydrofluoric acid poisoning," and at least two of them died in the process. Fluorine was only isolated in 1886, after almost a century of dangerous trying.

I was fascinated by reading this history, and immediately, recklessly, wanted to obtain fluorine for myself. Hydrofluoric acid was easy to get: Uncle Tungsten used vast quantities of it to "pearl" his lightbulbs, and I had seen great carboys of it in his factory in Hoxton. But when I told my parents the story of the fluorine martyrs, they forbade me to experiment with it in the house. (I compromised by keeping a small gutta-percha bottle of hydrofluoric acid in my lab, but my own fear of it was such that I never actually opened the bottle.)

It was really only later, when I thought about it, that I became astonished at the nonchalant way in which Griffin (and my other books) proposed the use of intensely poisonous substances. I had not the least difficulty getting potassium cyanide from the chemist's, the pharmacy, down the road—it was normally used for collecting insects in a killing bottle—but I could rather easily have killed myself with the stuff. I gathered, over a couple of years, a variety of chemicals that could have poisoned or blown up the entire street, but I was careful—or lucky.[3]

If my nose was stimulated in the lab by certain smells—the pungent, irritating smell of ammonia or sulfur dioxide, the odious smell of hydrogen sulfide—it was much more pleasantly stimulated by the garden outdoors and the kitchen, with its food smells, and its essences and spices, inside. What gave coffee its aroma? What were the essential substances

---

[3]Now, of course, none of these chemicals can be bought, and even school or museum laboratories are increasingly confined to reagents that are less hazardous—and less fun.

Linus Pauling, in an autobiographical sketch, described how he, too, obtained potassium cyanide (for a killing bottle) from a local druggist:

> Just think of the differences today. A young person gets interested in chemistry and is given a chemical set. But it doesn't contain potassium cyanide. It doesn't even contain copper sulfate or anything else interesting because all the interesting chemicals are considered dangerous substances. Therefore, these budding young chemists don't have a chance to do anything engrossing with their chemistry sets. As I look back, I think it is pretty remarkable that Mr. Ziegler, this friend of the family, would have so easily turned over one-third of an ounce of potassium cyanide to me, an eleven-year-old boy.

When I paid a visit not long ago to the old building in Finchley which had been Griffin & Tatlock's home a half century ago, it was no longer there. Such shops, such suppliers, which had provided chemicals and simple apparatus and unimaginable delights for generations, have now all but vanished.

in cloves, apples, roses? What gave onions and garlic and radishes their pungent smell? What, for that matter, gave rubber its peculiar odor? I especially liked the smell of hot rubber, which seemed to me to have a slightly human smell (both rubber and people, I learned later, contain odoriferous isoprene). Why did butter and milk acquire sour smells if they "went off," as they tended to do in hot weather? What gave "turps," oil of turpentine, its lovely, piney smell? Besides all these "natural" smells, there were the smells of the alcohol and acetone that my father used in the surgery, and of the chloroform and ether in my mother's obstetric bag. There was the gentle, pleasant, medical smell of iodoform, used to disinfect cuts, and the harsh smell of carbolic acid, used to disinfect lavatories (it carried a skull and crossbones on its label).

Scents could be distilled, it seemed, from all parts of a plant—leaves, petals, roots, bark. I tried to extract some fragrances by steam distillation, gathering rose petals and magnolia blossoms and grass cuttings from the garden and boiling them with water. Their essential oils would be volatilized in the steam and settle on top of the distillate as it cooled (the heavy, brownish essential oil of onions or garlic, though, would sink to the bottom). Alternatively one could use fat—butter fat, chicken fat—to make a fatty extract, a pomatum; or use solvents like acetone or ether. On the whole my extractions were not too successful, but I succeeded in making some reasonable lavender water, and extracting clove oil and cinnamon oil with acetone. The most productive extractions came from my visits to Hampstead Heath, when I gathered large bags of pine needles and made a fine, bracing green oil full of terpenes—the smell reminded me a little of the Friar's Balsam that I would be set to inhale, in steam, whenever I had a cold.

I loved the smell of fruits and vegetables and would savor everything, sniff at it, before I ate. We had a pear tree in the garden, and my mother would make a thick pear nectar from its fruit, in which the smell of pears seemed heightened. But the scent of pears, I had read, could be made artificially, too (as was done with "pear drops"), without using any pears. One had only to start with one of the alcohols—ethyl, methyl, amyl, whatever—and distill it with acetic acid to form the corresponding ester. I was amazed that something as simple as ethyl acetate could be responsible for the complex, delicious smell of pears, and that tiny chemical changes could transform this to other fruity scents—change the ethyl to isoamyl, and one had the smell of ripening apples; other small modifications would give esters that smelled of bananas or apricots or pineapples or grapes. This was my first experience of the power of chemical synthesis.

There were, besides the pleasant fruity smells, a number of vile, animally smells that one could easily make from simple ingredients or extract from plants. Auntie Len, with her botanical knowledge, sometimes colluded with me here, and introduced me to a plant called stinking goosefoot, a species of *Chenopodium*. If this was distilled in an alkaline medium—I used soda—a particularly vile-smelling and volatile material came off, which stank of rotten crabs or fish. The volatile substance, trimethylamine, was surprisingly simple—I had thought the smell of rotting fish would have a more complex basis. In America, Len told me, they had a plant called skunk cabbage, and this contained compounds that smelled like corpses or putrefying flesh; I asked if she could get me some, but, perhaps fortunately, she could not.

Some of these stinks incited me to pranks. We would get fresh fish every Friday, carp and pike, which my mother would grind to make the gefilte fish for shabbas. One Friday I added a little trimethylamine to the fish, and when my mother smelled this, she grimaced and threw the lot away.

My interest in smells made me wonder how we recognized and categorized odors, how the nose could instantly delineate esters from aldehydes, or recognize a category such as terpenes, as it were, at a glance. Poor as our sense of smell was compared to a dog's—our dog, Greta, could detect her favorite foods if a tin was opened at the other end of the house—there nevertheless seemed in humans to be a chemical analyzer at work at least as sophisticated as the eye or the ear. There did not seem to be any simple order, like the scale of musical tones, or the colors of the spectrum; yet the nose was quite remarkable in making categorizations that corresponded, in some way, to the basic structure of the chemical molecules. All the halogens, while different, had halogenlike smells. Chloroform smelled exactly like bromoform and (while not identical) had the same sort of smell as carbon tetrachloride (sold as the dry-cleaning fluid Thawpit). Most esters were fruity; alcohols—the simplest ones, anyway—had similar "alcoholic" smells; and aldehydes and ketones, too, had their own characteristic smells.

(Errors, surprises, could certainly occur, and Uncle Dave told me how phosgene, carbonyl chloride, the terrible poison gas used in the First World War, instead of signaling its danger by a halogenlike smell, had a deceptive scent like new-mown hay. This sweet, rustic smell, redolent of the hayfields of their boyhood, was the last sensation phosgene-gassed soldiers had just before they died.)

The bad smells, the stenches, always seemed to come from compounds containing sulfur (the smells of garlic and onion were simple organic sulfides, as closely related chemically as they were botanically), and these reached their climax in the sulfuretted alcohols, the mercaptans. The smell of skunks was due to butyl mercaptan, I read—this was pleasant, refreshing, when very dilute, but appalling, overwhelming, at close quarters. (I was delighted, when I read *Antic Hay* a few years later, to find that Aldous Huxley had named one of his less delectable characters Mercaptan.)

Thinking of all the malodorous sulfur compounds and the atrocious smell of selenium and tellurium compounds, I decided that these three elements formed an olfactory as well as a chemical category, and thought of them thereafter as the "stinkogens."

I had smelled a bit of hydrogen sulfide in Uncle Dave's lab—it smelled of rotten eggs and farts and (I was told) volcanoes. A simple way of making it was to pour dilute hydrochloric acid on ferrous sulfide. (The ferrous sulfide, a great chunky mass of it, I made myself by heating iron and sulfur together till they glowed and combined.) The ferrous sulfide bubbled when I poured hydrochloric acid on it, and instantly emitted a huge quantity of stinking, choking hydrogen sulfide. I threw open the doors into the garden and staggered out, feeling very queer and ill, remembering how poisonous the gas was. Meanwhile, the infernal sulfide (I had made a lot of it) was still giving off clouds of toxic gas, and this soon permeated the house. My parents were, by and large, amazingly tolerant of my experiments, but they insisted, at this point, on having a fume cupboard installed and on my using, for such experiments, less generous quantities of reagents.

When the air had cleared, morally and physically, and the fume cupboard had been installed, I decided to make other gases, simple compounds of hydrogen with other elements besides sulfur. Knowing that selenium and tellurium were closely akin to sulfur, in the same chemical group, I employed the same basic formula: compounding the selenium or tellurium with iron, and then treating the ferrous selenide or ferrous telluride with acid. If the smell of hydrogen sulfide was bad, that of hydrogen selenide was a hundred times worse—an indescribably horrible, disgusting smell that caused me to choke and tear, and made me think of putrefying radishes or cabbage (I had a fierce hatred of cabbage and brussels sprouts at this time, for boiled, overboiled, they had been staples at Braefield).

Hydrogen selenide, I decided, was perhaps the worst smell in the world. But hydrogen telluride came close, was also a smell from hell. An up-to-date hell, I decided, would have not just rivers of fiery brimstone, but lakes of boiling selenium and tellurium, too.

Twenty-four years ago I entered the wards of Mount Carmel and met the remarkable post-encephalitic patients who had been immured there since the great *encephalitis lethargica* (sleeping sickness) epidemic just after the First World War. Von Economo, who first described the *encephalitis lethargica* half a century before, had spoken of the most affected patients as "extinct volcanoes." In the spring of 1969, in a way which he could not have imagined, which no one could have imagined or foreseen, these "extinct volcanoes" erupted into life. The placid atmosphere of Mount Carmel was transformed—occurring before us was a cataclysm of almost geological proportions, the explosive "awakening," the "quickening," of eighty or more patients who had long been regarded, and regarded themselves, as effectively dead. I cannot think back on this time without profound emotion—it was the most significant and extraordinary in my life, no less than in the lives of our patients. All of us at Mount Carmel were caught up with the emotion, the excitement, and with something akin to enchantment, even awe.

It was not a purely "medical" excitement, any more than these awakenings were a purely medical event. There was a tremendous *human* (even allegorical) excitement at seeing the "dead" awaken again—it was at this point that I conceived the title *Awakenings,* taken from Ibsen's *When We Dead Awaken*—at seeing lives which one had thought irremediably blighted suddenly bloom into a wonderful renewal, at seeing individuals in all their vitality and richness emerge from the almost cadaveric state where they had been frozen and hidden for decades. We had had inklings of the vivid personalities so long immured—but the full reality of these only emerged, indeed burst upon us, with our patients' awakenings.

I was exceedingly lucky to encounter such patients at such a time, in such working conditions. But they were not the only post-encephalitic patients in the world—there were, in the late '60s, still many thousands, some in large groups, in institutions all over the world. There was no major country *without* its complement of post-encephalitics. And yet *Awakenings* is the only existing account of such patients—their decades-long "sleep" and, then, their dramatic "awakening" in 1969.

I found this exceedingly peculiar at the time: why, I thought, were there not other accounts of what must be happening all over the world? Why, for example, was there not an *Awakenings* from Philadelphia, where I knew of a group of patients not so dissimilar to my own? Why not from London, where the Highlands Hospital housed the largest post-encephalitic colony in England?[1] Or from Paris or Vienna, where the disease first struck?

There is no single answer to this; there were many things that mitigated against the sort of description, the "biographic" approach, of *Awakenings*.

One factor that made *Awakenings* possible had to do with the nature of the *situation*. Mount Carmel is a chronic hospital, an asylum; and physicians in general avoid such hospitals, or visit them briefly, and leave as soon as they can. This was not always the case: in the last century, Charcot virtually lived in the Salpêtrière, and Hughlings-Jackson at the West Riding Asylum—the founders of neurology realized well that it was only in such hospitals that the depths and details of the profounder disorders could be explored and worked out. As a resident I myself had never been to a chronic hospital, and though I had seen a number of patients with post-encephalitic Parkinsonism and other problems in outpatient clinics, I had no idea how profound and strange the effects of post-encephalitic disease might be. I found coming to Mount Carmel, in 1966, a revelation. It was my first encounter with disease of a depth I had never seen, read of, or heard of, before. The medical literature on the sleeping sickness had virtually

---

[1] There was a short, statistical paper by Calne et al. (1969), describing a six-week trial of L-DOPA in some of the Highlands patients, but there were no *biographical* accounts of "awakenings" in these, or any other, patients.

come to a stop in 1935, so that the profounder forms of it, occurring later, had never been described. I would not have imagined it *possible* for such patients to exist; or, if they existed, to remain undescribed. For physicians do not go, and reports do not emerge, from the "lower reaches," these abysses of affliction, which are now (so to speak) beneath the notice of Medicine. Few doctors ever entered the halls and back wards of chronic hospitals and asylums, and few had the patience to listen and look, to penetrate the physiologies and predicaments of these increasingly inaccessible patients.

The "other" side, the good side, of chronic hospitals is that what staff they have may work and live in them for decades, may become extraordinarily close to their charges, the patients, get to know and love them, recognize, respect them, *as people.* So when I came to Mount Carmel I did not just encounter "eighty cases of post-encephalitic disease," but eighty individuals, whose inner lives and total being was (to a considerable extent) known to the staff, known in the vivid, concrete knowing of relationship, not the pallid, abstract knowing of medical knowledge. Coming to this community—a community of patients, but also of patients and staff—I found myself encountering the patients as individuals, whom I could less and less reduce to statistics or lists of symptoms.

And, of course, this was a unique *time* for the patients, and for all of us. It had been established in the late 1950s that the Parkinsonian brain was lacking in the transmitter dopamine, and that it might therefore be "normalized" if the level of dopamine could be raised. But attempts to do this, by giving L-DOPA (a precursor of dopamine) in milligram quantities, had failed persistently—until Dr. George Cotzias, with great audacity, gave a group of patients L-DOPA in doses of a *thousand times* greater than had ever been used. With the publication of Cotzias's results in February 1967, the outlook for Parkinsonian patients was changed at a stroke: a sudden, unbelievable hope appeared—that patients hitherto able to look forward only to miserable and increasing disability might be (if not cured) transformed by the new drug. Life opened out once again, in imagination, for all our patients. For the first time in forty years they could believe in a future. The atmosphere from this time on was electric with excitement. One of the patients, Leonard L., when he heard of L-DOPA, rapped on his letterboard with mixed enthusiasm and irony, "Dopamine is Resurrectamine. Cotzias is the Chemical Messiah."

Yet it was not L-DOPA, or what it offered, which was so exciting for me when I first came as a young doctor, a year out of residency, to Mount Carmel. What excited me then was the spectacle of a disease that was never the same in two patients, a disease that could take any possible form—one rightly called a "phantasmagoria" by those who first studied it. ("There is nothing in the literature of medicine," wrote McKenzie in 1927, "to compare with the phantasmagoria of disorder manifested in the course of this strange malady.") At this level of the fantastic, the phantasmagoric, the encephalitis was enthralling. Much more fundamentally, it was, by virtue of the enormous range of disturbances occurring at every level of the nervous system, a disorder that could show, far better than any other, how the nervous system was organized, how brain and behavior, at their more primitive levels, worked. The biologist, the naturalist, in me was enthralled by all this—and led me to start gathering data at this time for a book on primitive, subcortical behaviors and controls.

But then, over and above the disorder, and its direct effects, were all the responses of the patients to their sickness—so what confronted one, what one studied, was not just disease or physiology, but *people,* struggling to adapt and survive. This too was clearly realized by the early observers, above all Ivy McKenzie: "The physician is concerned (unlike the naturalist) . . . with a single organism, the human subject, striving to preserve its identity in adverse circumstances." In perceiving this, I became something more than a naturalist (without, however, ceasing to be one). There evolved a new concern, a new bond: that of commitment to the patients, the individuals under my care. Through them I would explore what it was like to be human, to *stay* human, in the face of unimaginable adversities and threats. Thus, while continually monitoring their organic nature—their complex, ever-changing pathophysiologies and biologies—my central study and concern became *identity*—their struggle to maintain identity—to observe this, to assist this, and, finally, to describe this. All this was at the junction of biology and biography.

This sense of the dynamics of illness and life, of the

organism or subject striving to survive, sometimes under the strangest and darkest circumstances, was not a viewpoint which had been emphasized when I was a student or resident, nor was it one I found in the current medical literature. But when I saw these post-encephalitic patients, it was clearly and overwhelmingly true—indeed, it was the only way in which I *could* view them. Thus what had been dismissed disparagingly by most of my colleagues ("chronic hospitals—you'll never see anything interesting in *those* places") revealed itself as the complete opposite: an ideal situation in which to observe, to care, to explore. *Awakenings* would have been written, I think, even if there had not been any "awakening": it would then have been *People of the Abyss* (or *Cinquante Ans de Sommeil,* as the French edition has it), a delineation of the stillness and darkness of these arrested and frozen lives, and of the courage and humor with which patients, nonetheless, faced life.

The intensity of feeling for these patients, and equally of intellectual interest and curiosity about them, bound us together as a community at Mount Carmel; and this intensity rose to a peak in 1969, the actual year of the patients' "awakenings." In the spring of that year, I moved to an apartment a hundred yards from the hospital and would sometimes spend twelve or fifteen hours a day with our patients. I was with the patients constantly—I grudged the hours of sleep—observing them, talking with them, getting them to keep notebooks, and keeping voluminous notes myself, thousands of words each day. And if I had a pen in one hand, I had a camera in the other: I was seeing such things as had never, perhaps, been seen before—and which, in all probability, would never be seen again; it was my duty, and my joy, to record and bear witness. Many others also dedicated themselves, spent countless hours in the hospital. All of us involved with the patients—nurses, social workers, therapists of every sort—were in constant communication: talking to each other excitedly in the passage, phoning each other on weekends and at night, constantly exchanging new experiences and ideas. The excitement, the enthusiasm, of that year was remarkable; *this,* it seems to me, was an essential part of the *Awakenings* experience.

And yet, at the start, I scarcely knew what to expect. I had read the half-dozen reports on L-DOPA published in 1967 and '68, but felt my own patients to be very different. They did not have ordinary Parkinson's disease (like the other patients reported), but a post-encephalitic disorder of far greater complexity, severity, and strangeness. How would *these* patients, with their so-different disease, react? I felt I had to be cautious—almost exaggeratedly so. When, early in 1969, I embarked on the work which was later to become *Awakenings,* I conceived it in quite limited and narrowly "scientific" terms—as a ninety-day, double-blind trial of L-DOPA in a large group of patients who had become institutionalized after having encephalitis. L-DOPA was considered an experimental drug at this time, and I needed to get (from the Food and Drug Administration) a special investigator's license to use it. It was a condition of such licenses that one use "orthodox" methods, including a double-blind trial, coupled with presentation of results in quantitative form.

But it became obvious within a month or less that the original format would have to be abandoned. The effects of L-DOPA in these patients was decisive—spectacular; while, as I could infer from the precise 50 percent failure rate, there was no significant placebo effect whatever. I could no longer, in good conscience, continue the placebo but had to try L-DOPA in every patient; and I could no longer think of giving it for ninety days and then stopping—this would have been like stopping the very air that they breathed. Thus what was originally conceived as a limited ninety-day experiment was transformed instead into a historical experience: a story, in effect, of life for these patients as it had been before L-DOPA, and as it was changed, and as it was to become, after starting treatment with L-DOPA.

Thus I was impelled, willy-nilly, to a presentation of case-histories or biographies, for no "orthodox" presentation, in terms of numbers, series, grading effects, etc., could have conveyed the historical reality of the experience. In August 1969, then, I wrote the first nine case histories, or "stories," of *Awakenings.*

The same impulse, the same sense that one had to convey stories and phenomena—the drama of stories, the delight of phenomena—led me to write a number of letters to the editor, which I dispatched to the *Lancet* and the *British Medical Journal* early the next year. I enjoyed writing these letters, and as far as I could gather, readers of these

journals enjoyed reading them too. There was something
about their format and style that allowed me to convey the
wonder of the clinical experience, in a way that would
have been quite impossible in a medical article.

I now decided to present my overall observations, and
my general conclusions, while still adhering to an episto-
lary format. My earlier letters to the *Lancet* had been anec-
dotal (and everyone loves anecdotes); I had not yet
attempted any general formulations. My first experiences,
the patients' first responses, in the summer of '69, had
been happy ones; there had been an astonishing, festive
"awakening," at the time—but then all of my patients ran
into trouble and tribulation. I observed, at this time, not
only specific "side-effects" of L-DOPA, but certain *general*
patterns of trouble—sudden and unpredictable fluctuations
of response, the rapid development of oscillations, the
development of extreme sensitivity to L-DOPA, and finally,
the absolute impossibility of matching dose and effect—all
of which I found dismaying in the extreme. I tried altering
the dose of L-DOPA, but this no longer worked—the "system" now seemed to have a dynamic of its own.

In the summer of 1970, then, in a letter to the *Journal of
the American Medical Association,* I reported these findings,
describing the total effects of L-DOPA in sixty patients whom
I had maintained on it for a year. *All* of these, I noted, had
done well at first; but all of them, sooner or later, had
escaped from control, had entered complex, sometimes
bizarre, and unpredictable states. These could not, I indi-
cated, be seen as "side effects," but had to be seen as inte-

gral parts of an evolving whole. Ordinary considerations and policies, I stressed, sooner or later ceased to work. There was a need for a deeper, more radical understanding.

My *JAMA* letter caused a furor among some of my colleagues. I was astonished and shocked by the storm that blew up; and, in particular, by the tone of some of the letters. Some colleagues insisted that such effects "never" occurred; others that, even if they did, the matter should be kept quiet, lest it disturb "the atmosphere of therapeutic optimism needed for the maximal efficiency of L-DOPA." It was even thought, absurdly, that I was "against" L-DOPA—but it was not L-DOPA but reductionism that I was against. I invited my colleagues to come to Mount Carmel, to see for themselves the reality of what I had reported; none of them took up my invitation. I had not properly realized, until this time, the power of *wish* to distort and deny—and its prevalence in this complex situation, where the enthusiasm of doctors, and the distress of patients, might lie in unconscious collusion, equally concerned to wish away an unpalatable truth. The situation had similarities to what had occurred twenty years before, when cortisone was clothed with unlimited promise; and one could only hope that with the passage of time, and the accumulation of undeniable experience, a sense of reality would triumph over wish.

Was my letter too condensed—or simply confusing? Did I need to put things in the form of extended articles? With much labor (because it went against the grain, so to speak), I put everything I could in an orthodox or conventional format—papers full of statistics and figures and tables and graphs—and submitted these to various medical and neurological journals. To my amazement and chagrin, none was accepted—some of them, indeed, elicited vehemently censorious, even violent, rejections, as if there were something intolerable in what I had written. This confirmed my feeling that a deep nerve had been struck, that I had somehow elicited not just a medical, but a sort of epistemological, anxiety—and rage.[2]

I had not only cast doubt on what had appeared at first to be the extremely simple matter of giving a drug and being in control of its effects; I had cast doubt on predictability itself. I had (perhaps without fully realizing it myself) hinted at something bizarre, a contradiction of ordinary ways of thinking, and of the ordinary, accepted pic-

---

[2]Five years later, it happened that one of the neurologists who had taken such exception to my letter in *JAMA*—he had said that my observations were beyond credibility—found himself chairing a meeting at which the documentary film of *Awakenings* was being shown. There is a particular point in the film at which various bizarre "side effects" and instabilities of drug reaction are shown in dizzying array, and I was fascinated to observe my colleague's reactions here. First, he stared amazed, and his mouth dropped open; it was as if he were seeing such things for the first time, and his reaction was one of innocent and almost childlike wonder. Then he flushed a dark and angry crimson—whether with embarrassment or mortification, I could not tell; these were the very things he had dismissed as "beyond credibility," and now he was being forced to see them for himself. Then he developed a curious *tic,* a convulsive movement of the head which kept turning it away from the screen he could no longer bear to see. Then, finally, with great abruptness and violence, and muttering to himself, he burst out of his seat, in midfilm, and rushed out of the room. I found this behavior extraordinary and instructive, for it showed how profound, how utterly overwhelming, reactions to the "incredible" and "intolerable" might be.

ture of the world. A specter of extreme oddness, of radical contingency, had come up—and all this was disquieting, confounding, in the extreme ("These things are so bizarre that I cannot bear to contemplate them"—-Poincaré).

And so, by mid-1970 I was brought to a halt, at least so far as any publication was concerned. The work continued, full of excitement, unabated, and I accumulated (I dared to think) an absolute treasure of observations and of hypotheses and reflections associated with them, but I had no idea what to do with them. I knew that I had been given the rarest of opportunities; I knew that I had something valuable to say; but I saw no way of saying it, of being faithful to my experiences, without forfeiting medical "publishability" or acceptance among my colleagues. This was a time of great bewilderment and frustration, considerable anger, and sometimes despair.

This impasse was broken in September of 1972, when the editor of *The Listener* invited me to write an article on my experiences. This was going to be my opportunity. Instead of the censorious rejections I was used to, I was actually being invited to write, being offered a chance to publish, fully and freely, what had been accumulating and building up, dammed up, for so long. I wrote "The Great Awakening" at a single sitting—neither I nor the editor altered a single word—and it was published the following month. Here, with a sense of great liberation from the constraints of "medicalizing" and medical jargon, I described the wonderful panorama of phenomena I had seen in my patients. I described the raptures of their "awakenings," I described the torments that so often followed; but above all, it was *phenomena* which I was concerned to describe, with a neutral and phenomenological (rather than a therapeutic, or "medical") eye.

But the picture, the theory, implied by the phenomena: this seemed to me to be of a revolutionary sort—"a new neurophysiology," as I wrote, "of a quantum-relativistic sort." These were bold words indeed; they excited me, and others—although I soon came to think that I had said too much, and too little. That there was *something,* assuredly, very strange going on—not quantality, not relativity, but something much commoner, yet stranger. I could not imagine what this was, in 1972, though it haunted me when I came to complete *Awakenings,* and rippled through it constantly, evasively, as half-tantalizing metaphors.

The article in *The Listener* was followed (in contrast to the hateful *JAMA* experience of two years earlier) by a wave of interest, and a great number of letters, an exciting correspondence which lasted several weeks. This response put an end to my long years of frustration and obstruction and gave me a decisive encouragement and affirmation. I picked up my long discarded case-histories of 1969, added eleven more, and in two weeks completed *Awakenings.* The case-histories were the easiest to write; they wrote themselves, they stemmed straight from experience, and I have always regarded them with especial affection as the true and unassailable center of *Awakenings.* The rest is disputable, the stories are so.

But the 1973 publication of *Awakenings,* while attracting much general attention, met the same cold reception from the profession as my articles had done earlier. There was not a single medical notice or review, only a disapproving or uncomprehending silence. There was one brave editor (of the *British Clinical Journal*) who spoke out on this, making *Awakenings* his "editor's choice" for 1973, but commenting on "the strange mutism" of the profession toward it.

I was devastated at this medical "mutism," but at the same time reassured and encouraged by the reaction of A. R. Luria. Luria himself, after a lifetime of minute neuropsychological observations, had himself published two extraordinary, almost novelistic case histories—*The Mind of a Mnemonist* (in 1968) and *The Man with a Shattered World* (1972). To my intense pleasure, in the strange medical silence which attended the publication of *Awakenings,* I received a letter, two letters, from him; in the first, he spoke of his own "biographic" books and approaches:

> Frankly said, I myself like very much the type of "biographical" study, such as Sherashevsky [the Mnemonist] and Zazetski [the man with the "shattered world"] . . . firstly because it is a kind of "Romantic Science" which I wanted to introduce, partly because I am strongly *against* a formal statistical approach and *for* a qualitative study of personality, *for* every attempt to find *factors* underlying the structure of personality. [Letter of July 19, 1973, emphasis in original]

And in the second, he spoke of *Awakenings:*

I received *Awakenings* and have read it at once with great
delight. I was ever conscious and sure that a good clinical
description of cases plays a leading role in medicine, especially in Neurology and Psychiatry. Unfortunately, the
ability to describe which was so common to the great
Neurologists and Psychiatrists of the 19th century [is] lost
now, perhaps because of the basic mistake that mechanical
and electrical devices can replace the study of personality. . . . Your excellent book shows, that the important tradition of clinical case studies can be revived and with a
great success. [Letter of July 25, 1973]

He then went on to ask me some specific questions,
above all expressing his fascination that L-DOPA should be
so various and unstable in effect.[3]

I had admired Luria infinitely since my medical school
days, and before. When I heard him lecture in London in

---

[3]He returned to this topic the following month, when he said that he had been
fascinated by the case of Martha N., and the fact that she had responded to
L-DOPA in six different ways: "*Why* was it different each time?" he asked, "*Why*
could one not replay things again and again?"—questions I could not answer
in 1973. It seemed to me typical of the genius of Luria that he had at once
homed in on one of the central mysteries and challenges of *Awakenings*—the
various and unrepeatable and unpredictable character of patients' responses—
and been fascinated by this; whereas my neurological colleagues, by and large,
had been frightened and dismayed by this, had tended to asseverate, "It's not
so, it's not so."

1959, I was overwhelmed by his combination of intellectual power and human warmth—I had often encountered these separately, but I had not too often encountered them *together*—and it was exactly this combination which so pleased me in his work, and which made it such an antidote to certain trends in medical writing, which attempted to delete both subjectivity and reflection. Luria's early works had been, sometimes, a little stilted in character, but they grew in intellectual warmth, in wholeness, as he grew older, culminating in his two late works, *The Mind of a Mnemonist* and *The Man with a Shattered World*. I do not know how much either of these works influenced me, but they certainly emboldened me, and made it easier to write and publish *Awakenings*.

Luria often said that he had to write two sorts of books, wholly different but wholly complementary: "classical," analytic texts (like *Higher Cortical Functions in Man*) and "romantic," biographical books (like *The Mind of a Mnemonist* and *The Man with a Shattered World*). I was also conscious of this double need, and found there were always *two* books, potentially, demanded by every clinical experience: one more purely "medical" or "classical"—an objective description of disorders, mechanisms, syndromes; the other more existential and personal—an emphatic entering into patients' experiences and worlds. Two such books dawned in me when I first saw our post-encephalitic patients: *Compulsion and Constraint* (a study of subcortical disorders and mechanisms) and *People of the Abyss* (a novelish, Jack Londonish book). They only came together, finally, in 1969—

in a book which tried to be *both* classical and romantic; to place itself at the intersection of biology and biography; to combine, as best it could, the modes of paradigm and art.

But *no* model, finally, seemed to suit my requirements—for what I was seeing, and what I needed to convey, was neither purely classical nor purely romantic, but seemed to move into the profound realm of allegory or myth. Even my title, *Awakenings,* had a double meaning, partly literal, partly in the mode of metaphor or myth.

The elaborate case history, the "romantic" style, with its endeavor to present a whole life, the repercussions of a disease, in all its richness, had fallen very much out of favor by the middle of the century—and this, perhaps, was one reason for the "strange mutism" of the profession when *Awakenings* was first published in 1973. But as the seventies progressed, this antipathy to case-history diminished—it even became possible (though difficult) to publish case histories in the medical literature. With this thawing of atmosphere, there was a renewed sense that complex neural and psychic functions (and their disorders) *required* detailed and nonreductive narratives for their explication and understanding.[4]

At the same time, the unpredictable responses to L-DOPA I saw with my patients in 1969—their sudden fluctua-

---

[4]There has been a parallel movement in anthropology since 1970—this had also been becoming meager and mechanical—with a new, or renewed, insistence on what Clifford Geertz has dubbed "thick" description.

tions and oscillations, their extraordinary "sensitization" to L-DOPA, to *everything*—were now being seen, increasingly, by everyone. Post-encephalitic patients, it became clear, might show these bizarre reactions within weeks, sometimes days—whereas "ordinary" Parkinsonian patients, with their more stable nervous systems, might not show them for several years. Yet, sooner or later, *all* patients maintained on L-DOPA started to show these strange, unstable states—and with the FDA approval of L-DOPA in 1970, their numbers mounted, finally to millions. And now, everybody found the same: the central promise of L-DOPA was confirmed, a million-fold—but so too was the central threat, the certainty of "side effects" or "tribulations," sooner or later.

Thus what had been surprising or intolerable when I first published *Awakenings* was—by the time the third edition was published in 1982—confirmed for all my colleagues by their own, undeniable experience. The optimistic and irrational mood of the early days of L-DOPA had changed to something more sober and realistic. This mood, well established by 1982, made the new edition of *Awakenings* acceptable, and even a classic, to my medical colleagues, where the original had been unacceptable nine years before.

It is the imagination of other people's worlds—worlds almost inconceivably strange, yet inhabited by people just like ourselves, people, indeed, who might *be* ourselves—that forms the center of *Awakenings*. Other worlds, other lives, even though so different from our own, have the power of arousing the sympathetic imagination, of awakening an intense and often creative resonance in others. We may never have seen a Rose R., but once we have read of her we see the world differently—we can imagine her world, with a sort of awe, and with this our world is suddenly enlarged. A wonderful example of such a creative response was given by Harold Pinter in his play, *A Kind of Alaska;* this is Pinter's world, the landscape of his unique gifts and sensibility, but it is also Rose R.'s world, and the world of *Awakenings*. Pinter's play has been followed by several adaptations of *Awakenings* for stage and screen; each of these has drawn on different aspects of the book. Every reader will bring to *Awakenings* his own imagination and sensibilities, and will find, if he lets himself, his world strangely deepened, imbued with a new depth of tenderness and perhaps horror. For these patients, while seemingly so extraordinary, so "special," have in them something of the universal, and can call to everyone, awaken everyone, as they called to and awakened me.

I hesitated very greatly in regard to the original publication of our patients' "story" and their lives. But they themselves encouraged me, and said to me from the first, "Tell our story—or it will never be known."

A few of the patients are still alive—we have known each other for twenty-four years now. But those who have died are in some sense not dead—their unclosed charts, their letters, still face me as I write. They still live, for me, in some very personal way. They were not only patients but teachers and friends, and the years I spent with them were the most significant of my life. I want something of their lives, their presence, to be preserved and live for others, as exemplars of human predicament and survival. This is the testimony, the only testimony, of a unique event—but one which may become an allegory for us all.

# ROSE R.

Miss R. was born in New York City in 1905, the youngest child of a large, wealthy, and talented family. Her childhood and school days were free of serious illness, and were marked, from their earliest days, by love of merriment, games, and jokes. High-spirited, talented, full of interests and hobbies, sustained by deep family affection and love, and a sure sense of who and what and why she was, Miss R. steered clear of significant neurotic problems or "identity-crises" in her growing-up period.

On leaving school, Miss R. threw herself ardently into a social and peripatetic life. Airplanes, above all, appealed to her eager, volant, and irrepressible spirit; she flew to Pittsburgh and Denver, New Orleans and Chicago, and twice to the California of Hearst and Hollywood (no mean feat in the planes of those days). She went to innu-

merable parties and shows, was toasted and fêted, and
rolled home drunk at night. And between parties and
flights she dashed off sketches of the bridges and water-
fronts with which New York abounded. Between 1922
and 1926, Miss R. lived in the blaze of her own vitality,
and lived more than most other people in the whole of
their lives. And this was as well, for at the age of twenty-
one she was suddenly struck down by a virulent form of
*encephalitis lethargica*—one of its last victims before the epidemic vanished. Nineteen twenty-six, then, was the last
year in which Miss R. really *lived*.

The night of the sleeping sickness, and the days which
followed it, can be reconstructed in great detail from
Miss R.'s relatives, and Miss R. herself. The acute phase
announced itself (as sometimes happened: compare Maria
G.) by nightmares of a grotesque and terrifying and pre-
monitory nature. Miss R. had a series of dreams about one
central theme: she dreamed she was imprisoned in an
inaccessible castle, but the castle had the form and shape
of herself; she dreamed of enchantments, bewitchments,
entrancements; she dreamed that she had become a living,
sentient statue of stone; she dreamed that the world had
come to a stop; she dreamed that she had fallen into a sleep
so deep that nothing could wake her; she dreamed of a
death which was different from death. Her family had difficulty waking her the next morning, and when she awoke
there was intense consternation: "Rose," they cried,
"wake up! What's the matter? Your expression, your posi-

tion . . . You're so still and so strange." Miss R. could not answer, but turned her eyes to the wardrobe mirror, and there she saw that her dreams had come true. The local doctor was brisk and unhelpful: "Catatonia," he said; *"Flexibilitas cerea.* What can you expect with the life she's been leading? She's broken her heart over one of these bums. Keep her quiet and feed her—she'll be fine in a week."

But Miss R. was not to recover for a week, or a year, or forty-three years. She recovered the ability to speak in short sentences, or to make sudden movements before she froze up again. She showed, increasingly, a forced retraction of her neck and her eyes—a state of almost continuous oculogyric crisis, broken only by sleep, meals, and occasional "releases." She was alert, and seemed to notice what went on around her; she lost none of her affection for her numerous family—and they lost none of their affection for her; but she seemed absorbed and preoccupied in some unimaginable state. For the most part, she showed no sign of distress, and no sign of anything save intense *concentration:* "She looked," said one of her sisters, "as if she were trying her hardest to remember something—or, maybe, doing her damnedest to forget something. Whatever it was, it took all her attention." In her years at home, and subsequently in hospital, her family did their utmost to penetrate this absorption, to learn what was going on with their beloved "kid" sister. With them—and, much later, with me—Miss R. was exceedingly candid, but whatever she said seemed cryptic and gnomic, and yet at the same time disquietingly clear.[1]

---

[1] I would often ask Miss R. what she was thinking about.

"Nothing, just nothing," she would say.

"But how can you possibly be thinking of nothing?"

"It's dead easy, once you know how."

"*How* exactly do you think about nothing?"

"One way is to think about the same thing again and again. Like $2 = 2 = 2 = 2$; or, I am what I am what I am what I am. . . . It's the same thing with my posture. My posture continually leads to itself. Whatever I do or whatever I think leads deeper and deeper into itself. . . . And then there are maps."

"Maps? What do you mean?"

"Everything I do is a map of itself, everything I do is a part of itself. Every part leads into itself. . . . I've got a thought in my mind, and then I see something in it, like a dot on the skyline. It comes nearer and nearer, and then I see what it is—it's just the same thought I was thinking before. And then I see another dot, and another, and so on. . . . Or I think of a map; then a map of that map; then a map of that map of that map, and each map perfect, though smaller and smaller. . . . Worlds within worlds within worlds within worlds. . . . Once I get going I can't possibly stop. It's like being caught between mirrors, or echoes, or something. Or being caught on a merry-go-round which won't come to a stop."

Sometimes, Miss R. told me, she would feel compelled to circumscribe the sides of a mental quadrangle, a "paddock" composed of seven notes of an endlessly reiterated Verdi aria: *"Tum—*ti-*tum—*ti-*tum—*ti-*tum,"* a forced mental perambulation which might go on for hours or days. And at other times she would be forced to "travel," mentally, through an endless 3-D tunnel of intersecting lines, the end of the tunnel rushing toward her but never reached.

"And do you have any *other* ways of thinking about nothing, Rosie?"

"Oh yes! The dots and maps are *positive* nothings, but I also think of *negative* nothings."

"And what are those like?"

"That's impossible to say, because they're takings-away. I think of a thought, and it's suddenly gone—like having a picture whipped out of its frame. Or I try to picture something in my mind, but the picture dissolves as fast as I can make it. I have a particular idea, but can't keep it in mind; and then I lose the *general* idea; and then the general idea *of* a general idea; and in two or three jumps my mind is a blank—*all* my thoughts gone, blanked out or erased."

When there was only this state, and no other problems, Miss R.'s family could keep her at home: she was no trouble, they loved her, she was simply—elsewhere (or nowhere). But three or four years after her trance-state had started, she started to become rigid on the left side of her body, to lose her balance when walking, and to develop other signs of Parkinsonism. Gradually these symptoms grew worse and worse, until full-time nursing became a necessity. Her siblings left home, and her parents were aging, and it was increasingly difficult to keep her at home. Finally, in 1935, she was admitted to Mount Carmel.

Her state changed little after the age of thirty, and when I first saw her in 1966, my findings coincided with the original notes from her admission. Indeed, the old staff-nurse on her ward, who had known her throughout, said: "It's uncanny, that woman hasn't aged a day in the thirty years I've known her. The rest of us get older—but Rosie's the same." It was true: Miss R. at sixty-one looked thirty years younger; she had raven-black hair, and her face was unlined, as if she had been magically preserved by her trance or her stupor.

She sat upright and motionless in her wheelchair, with little or no spontaneous movement for hours on end. There was no spontaneous blinking, and her eyes stared straight ahead, seemingly indifferent to her environment but completely absorbed. Her gaze, when requested to look in different directions, was full, save for complete inability to converge the eyes. Fixation of gaze lacked smooth and subtle modulation, and was accomplished by sudden, gross movements which seemed to cost her considerable effort. Her face was completely masked and expressionless. The tongue could not be protruded beyond the lip-margins, and its movements, on request, were exceedingly slow and small. Her voice was virtually inaudible, though Miss R. could whisper quite well with considerable effort. Drooling was profuse, saturating a cloth bib within an hour, and the entire skin was oily, seborrhoeic, and sweating intensely. Akinesia was global, although rigidity and dystonia were strikingly unilateral in distribution. There was intense axial rigidity, no movement of the neck or trunk muscles being possible. There was equally intense rigidity in the left arm, and a very severe dystonic contracture of the left hand. No voluntary movement of this limb was possible. The right arm was much less rigid, but showed great akinesia, all movements being minimal, and decaying to zero after two or three repetitions. Both legs were hypertonic, the left much more so. The left foot was bent inward in dystonic inversion. Miss R. could not rise to her feet unaided, but when assisted to do so could maintain her balance and take a few small, shuffling, precarious steps, although the tendency to backward-falling and pulsion was very great.

She was in a state of near-continuous oculogyric crisis, although this varied a good deal in severity. When it became more severe, her Parkinsonian "background" was increased in intensity, and an intermittent coarse tremor appeared in her right arm. Prominent tremor of the head, lips, and tongue also became evident at these times, and rhythmic movement of buccinators and corrugators. Her breathing would become somewhat stertorous at such times, and would be accompanied by a guttural phonation reminiscent of a pig grunting. Severe crises would always be accompanied by tachycardia and hypertension. Her neck would be thrown back in an intense and sometimes agonizing opisthotonic posture. Her eyes would generally stare directly ahead, and could not be moved by voluntary effort: in the severest crises they were forced upward and fixed on the ceiling.

Miss R.'s capacity to speak or move, minimal at the best of times, would disappear almost entirely during her severer crises, although in her greatest extremity she would some-times call out, in a strange high-pitched voice, perseverative and palilalic, utterly unlike her husky "normal" whisper: "Doctor, doctor, doctor, doctor . . . help me, help, help, h'lp, h'lp. . . . I am in terrible pain, I'm so frightened, so frightened, so frightened. . . . I'm going to die, I know it, I know it, I know it, I know it. . . ." And at other times, if nobody was near, she would whimper softly to herself, like some small animal caught in a trap. The nature of Miss R.'s pain during her crises was only elucidated later, when speech had become easy: some of it was a local pain associ-ated with extreme opisthotonos, but a large component seemed to be central—diffuse, unlocalizable, of sudden onset and offset, and inseparably coalesced with feelings of dread and threat, in the severest crises a true *angor animi*.

During exceptionally severe attacks, Miss R.'s face would become flushed, her eyes reddened and protruding, and she would repeat, "It'll kill me, it'll kill me, it'll kill me . . ." hundreds of times in succession.[2]

Miss R.'s state scarcely changed between 1966 and 1969, and when L-DOPA became available I was in two minds about using it. She was, it was true, intensely disabled, and had been virtually helpless for over forty years. It was her *strangeness* above all which made me hesitate and wonder—fearing what might happen if I gave her L-DOPA. I had never seen a patient whose regard was so turned away from the world, and so immured in a private, inaccessible world of her own.

I kept thinking of something Joyce wrote about his mad daughter: ". . . fervently as I desire her cure, I ask myself what then will happen when and if she finally withdraws her regard from the lightning-lit reverie of her clairvoyance and turns it upon that battered cabman's face, the world. . . ."

---

[2]Compare cases cited by Jelliffe: the patient who would cry out in "anguish" during her attacks, but could give no reason for her fear, or the patient who would feel every attack to be "a calamity" (see Jelliffe, 1932, pp. 36–42). The same term was often used by Lillian W., especially in relation to those very complex oculogyric crises which she sometimes called "humdingers." Even though she had oculogyric crises every week, she would invariably say during each attack, "This is the worst one I ever had. The others were just bad—*this* is a calamity." When I would remonstrate, "But Mrs. W., this is exactly what you said last week!" she would say, "I know. I was wrong. This one *is* a calamity." She never got used to her crises in the least—even though she had had them, each Wednesday, for more than forty years.

But I started her on L-DOPA, despite my misgivings, on June 18, 1969. The following is an extract from my diary.

*25 June.* The first therapeutic responses have already occurred, even though the dosage has only been raised to 1.5 gm. a day. Miss R. has experienced two entire days unprecedentedly free of oculogyric crises, and her eyes, so still and preoccupied before, are brighter and more mobile and attentive to her surroundings.

*1 July.* Very real improvements are evident by this date: Miss R. is able to walk unaided down the passage, shows a distinct reduction of rigidity in the left arm and elsewhere, and has become able to speak at a normal conversational volume. Her mood is cheerful, and she has had no oculogyric crises for three days. In view of this propitious response, and the absence of any adverse effects, I am increasing the dosage of L-DOPA to 4 gm. daily.

*6 July.* Now receiving 4 gm. L-DOPA. Miss R. has continued to improve in almost every way. When I saw her at lunchtime, she was delighted with everything: "Dr. Sacks!" she called out, "I walked to and from the new building today" (this is a distance of about six hundred yards). "It's fabulous, it's gorgeous!" Miss R. has now been free from oculogyric crises for eight days, and has shown no akathisia or undue excitement. I too feel delighted at her progress, but for some reason am conscious of obscure forebodings.

*7 July.* Today Miss R. has shown her first signs of unstable and abrupt responses to L-DOPA. Seeing her 3½ hours after her early-morning dose, I was shocked to find her very "down"—hypophonic, somewhat depressed, rigid and akinetic, with extremely small pupils and profuse salivation. Fifteen minutes after receiving her medication she was "up" again—her voice and walking fully restored, cheerful, smiling, talkative, her eyes alert and shining, and her pupils somewhat dilated. I was further disquieted by observing an occasional impulsion to run, although this was easily checked by her.

*8 July.* Following an insomniac night ("I didn't feel in the least sleepy: thoughts just kept rushing through my head"), Miss R. is extremely active, cheerful, and affectionate. She seems to be very busy, constantly flying from one place to another, and all her thoughts too are concerned with movement; "Dr. Sacks," she exclaimed breathlessly, "I feel great today. I feel I want to fly. I love you, Dr. Sacks, I love you, I love you. You know, you're the kindest doctor in the world. . . . You know I always liked to travel around: I used to fly to Pittsburgh, Chicago, Miami, California. . . ." etc. Her skin is warm and flushed, her pupils are again very widely dilated, and her eyes constantly glancing to and fro. Her energy seems limitless and untiring, although I get the impression of exhaustion somewhere beneath the pressured surface. An entirely new symptom has also appeared today, a sudden quick movement of the right hand to the chin, which is repeated two or three times an hour. When I questioned Miss R. about this she said: "It's new, it's odd, it's strange, I never did it before. God knows why I do it. I just suddenly get an *urge,* like you suddenly got to sneeze or scratch yourself." Fearing the onset of akathisia or excessive emotional excitement, I have reduced the dosage of L–DOPA to 3 gm. daily.

*9 July.* Today Miss R.'s energy and excitement are unabated, but her mood has veered from elation to anxiety. She is impatient, touchy, and extremely demanding. She became much agitated in the middle of the day, asserting that seven dresses had been stolen from her closet, and that her purse had been stolen. She entertained dark suspicions of various fellow patients: no doubt they had been plotting this for weeks before. Later in the day, she discovered that her dresses were in fact in her closet in their usual position. Her paranoid recriminations instantly vanished: "Wow!" she said, "I must have imagined it all. I guess I better take myself in hand."

*14 July.* Following the excitements and changing moods of July 9, Miss R.'s state has become less pressured and hyperactive. She has been able to sleep, and has lost the tic-like "wiping" movements of her right hand. Unfortunately, after a two-week remission, her old enemy has reemerged, and she has experienced two severe oculogyric crises. I observed in these not only the usual staring, but a more bizarre symptom—captivation or enthrallment of gaze: in one of these crises she had been forced to stare at one of her fellow patients, and had felt her eyes "drawn" this way and that, following the movements of this patient around the ward. "It was uncanny," Miss R. said later. "My eyes were spellbound. I felt like I was bewitched or something, like a rabbit with a snake." During the periods of "bewitchment" or fascination, Miss R. had the feeling that her "thoughts had stopped," and that she could only think of one thing, the object of her gaze. If, on the other hand, her attention was distracted, the quality of thinking would suddenly change, the motionless fascination would be broken up, and she would experience instead "an absolute torrent of thoughts," rushing through her mind: these thoughts did not seem to be "her" thoughts, they were not what she wanted to think, they were "peculiar thoughts" which appeared "by themselves." Miss R. could not or would not specify the nature of these intrusive thoughts, but she was greatly frightened by the whole business: "These crises are different from the ones I used to get," she said. "They are worse. They are completely *mad!*"[3]

*25 July.* Miss R. has had an astonishing ten days, and has shown phenomena I never thought possible. Her mood has been joyous and elated, and very salacious. Her social behavior has remained impeccable, but she has developed an insatiable urge to sing songs and tell jokes, and has made very full use of our portable tape recorder. In the past few days, she has recorded innumerable songs of an astonishing

---

[3]Jelliffe cites many cases of oculogyric crises with fixation of gaze and attention, and also of crises with reiterative "autochthonous" thinking. Miss R. never vouchsafed the nature of the "mad" thoughts which came to her during her crises at this time, and one would suspect from the reticence that these thoughts were of an inadmissible nature, either sexual or hostile. Jelliffe refers to several patients who were compelled to think of "dirty things" during their crises, and to another patient who experienced during his crises "ideas of reference to which he pays no attention" (see Jelliffe, 1932, pp. 37–39). Miriam H. would have delusional erotic reminiscences whenever she had an oculogyric crisis.

lewdness, and reams of "light" verse all dating from the twenties. She is also full of anecdotes and allusions to "current" figures—to figures who were current in the mid-1920s. We have been forced to do some archival research, looking at old newspaper files in the New York Library. We have found that almost all of Miss R.'s allusions date to 1926, her last year of real life before her illness closed round her. Her memory is uncanny, considering she is speaking of so long ago. Miss R. wants the tape recorder, and nobody around; she stays in her room, alone with the tape recorder; she is looking at everyone as if they didn't exist. She is completely engrossed in her memories of the twenties, and is doing her best to not notice anything later. I suppose one calls this "forced reminiscence," or incontinent nostalgia.[4] But I also have the feeling that she feels her "past" as present, and that, perhaps it has never felt "past"

---

[4] I saw similar phenomena, and had similar thoughts, regarding another patient (Sam G.), whose story, alas, I didn't tell in the original *Awakenings* (though his face appears on the front cover of the 1976 edition). Sam used to be both a car buff and racing driver, bizarrely helped in the latter by his preternaturally quick reactions and his sudden, "frivolous" moves. He had to give it up around 1930 due to envelopment in a profound Parkinsonism. "Awakening," for him, had some of the "nostalgic" quality it had for Rose R. In particular, the moment he found himself "released" by L-DOPA, he started drawing cars. He drew constantly, with great speed, and was *obsessed* by his drawing; if we did not keep him well supplied with paper, he would draw on the walls, on table-cloths, on his bedsheets. His cars were accurate, authentic, and had an odd charm. When he was not drawing, he was talking, or writing—of "the old days" in the twenties when he was driving and racing—and this too was full of vividness and immediacy, minute, compelling, *living* detail. He would be completely transported as he drew, talked, or wrote, and spoke of "the old days" *as if they were now;* the days before 1930 were clearly much more present than the real now; he seemed, like Rose R., to be living (or reliving) the past, even

for her. Is it possible that Miss R. has never, in fact, moved on from the "past"? *Could she still be "in" 1926 forty-three years later? Is 1926 "now"?*[5]

---

though (like her) he was perfectly "oriented." He *knew* that it was 1969, that he was aging, ill, and in hospital, but felt (and *conveyed*) his racing youth of the twenties.

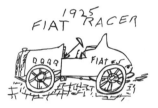

[5] When Rose did "awaken" with the administration of L-DOPA in 1969, she was extremely excited and animated, but in a way that was strange. She spoke of Gershwin and other contemporaries as if they were still alive; of events in the mid-twenties as if they had just happened. She had obsolete mannerisms and turns of speech; she gave the impression of a "flapper" come suddenly to life. We wondered if she was disoriented, if she knew where she was. I asked her various questions, and she gave me a succinct and chilling answer: "I can give you the date of Pearl Harbor," she said, "I can give you the date of Kennedy's assassination. I've registered it all—but none of it seems real. I *know* it's '69, I *know* I'm 64—but I *feel* it's '26, I *feel* I'm 21. I've been a spectator for the last forty-three years." (There were many other patients who behaved, and even appeared, much younger than their years, as if their personalities, their processes of personal growth and becoming, had been arrested at the same time as their other physical and mental processes.)

*Note (1990):* Edelman describes how consciousness and memory (which he sees as dependent on continual "recategorization") are, normally, continually "updated"; and how this updating depends, in the first place, on *movement,* on free and smooth and orderly movement. The basal ganglia are necessary for this—Edelman calls them "organs of succession." The absence of "updating" in Rose R., and in all our immobilized basal-ganglia–damaged patients, is in striking accordance with this notion.

*28 July*. Miss R. sought me out this morning—the first time she had done so in almost two weeks. Her face has lost its jubilant look, and she looks anxious and shadowed and slightly bewildered: "Things can't last," she said. "Something awful is coming. God knows what it is, but it's bad as they come." I tried to find out more, but Miss R. shook her head: "It's just a feeling, I can't tell you more. . . ."

*1 August*. A few hours after stating her prediction, Miss R. ran straight into a barrage of difficulties. Suddenly she was ticcing, jammed, and blocked; the beautiful smooth flow which had borne her along seemed to break up, and dam, and crash back on itself. Her walking and talking are gravely affected. She is impelled to rush forward for five or six steps, and then suddenly freezes or jams without warning; she continually gets more excited and frustrated, and with increasing excitement the jamming grows worse. If she can moderate her excitement or her impulsion to run, she can still walk the corridor without freezing or jamming. Analogous problems are affecting her speech: she can only speak softly, if she is to speak at all, for with increased vocal impetus she stutters and stops. I have the feeling that Miss R.'s "motor space" is becoming confined, so that she rebounds internally if she moves with too much speed or force. Reducing her L-DOPA to 3 gm. a day reduced the dangerous hurry and block, but led to an intensely severe oculogyric crisis—the worst Miss R. has had since starting L-DOPA. Moreover, her "wiping" tic—which reappeared on the 28th—has grown more severe and more *complex* with each passing hour. From a harmless feather-light brush of the chin, the movement has become a deep circular gouging, her right index finger scratching incessantly in tight little circles, abrading the skin and making it bleed. Miss R. has been quite unable to stop this compulsion *directly,* but she can override it by thrusting her tic-hand deep in her pocket and clutching its lining with all of her force. The moment she forgets to do this, the hand flies up and scratches her face.

## AUGUST 1969

During the first week of August,[6] Miss R. continued to have oculogyric crises every day of extreme severity, during which she would be intensely rigid and opisthotonic, anguished, whimpering, and bathed in sweat. Her tics of the right hand became almost too fast for the eye to follow, their rate having increased to almost three hundred per minute (an estimate confirmed by a slow-motion film). On August 6, Miss R. showed very obvious palilalia, repeating entire sentences and strings of words again and again: "I'm going round like a record," she said, "which gets stuck in the groove. . . ." During the second week of August, her tics became more complex, and were conflated with defensive maneuvers, counter-tics, and elaborate rituals. Thus Miss R. would clutch someone's hand, release her grip,

---

[6]The following is based on notes provided by our speech pathologist, Miss Marjorie Kohl. I myself was away during August.

touch something nearby, put her hand in her pocket, withdraw it, slap the pocket *three* times, put it back in the pocket, wipe her chin *five* times, clutch someone's hand . . . and move again and again through this stereotyped sequence.

The evening of August 15 provided the only pleasant interlude in a month otherwise full of disability and suffering. On this evening, quite unexpectedly, Miss R. emerged from her crises and blocking and ticcing, and had a brief return of joyous salacity, accompanied with free-flowing singing and movement. For an hour this evening, she improvised a variety of coprolalic limericks to the tune of "The Sheikh of Araby," accompanying herself on the piano with her uncontractured right hand.

Later this week, her motor and vocal block became absolute. She would suddenly call out to Miss Kohl: "Margie, I . . . Margie, I want . . . Margie! . . . ," completely unable to proceed beyond the first word or two of what she so desperately wanted to say. When she tried to write, similarly, her hand (and thoughts) suddenly stopped after a couple of words. If one asked her to try and say what she wanted, softly and slowly, her face would go blank, and her eyes would shift in a tantalized manner, indicating, perhaps, her frantic inner search for the dislimning thought. Walking became impossible at this time, for Miss R. would find her feet completely stuck to the ground, but the impulse to move would throw her flat on her face. During the last ten days of August, Miss R. seemed to be totally blocked in all spheres of activity; everything about her showed an extremity of tension, which was entirely prevented from finding any outlet. Her face at this time was continually clenched in a horrified, tortured, and anguished expression. Her prediction of a month earlier was completely fulfilled: something awful *had* come, and it was as bad as they came.

1969–72

Miss R.'s reactions to L-DOPA since the summer of 1969 have been almost nonexistent compared with her dramatic initial reaction. She has been placed on L-DOPA five further times, each with an increase of dose by degrees to about 3.0 gm. per day. Each time the L-DOPA has procured *some* reduction in her rigidity, oculogyria, and general entrancement, but less and less on each succeeding occasion. It has *never* called forth anything resembling the amazing mobility and mood change of July 1969, and in particular has never recalled the extraordinary sense of 1926-ness which she had at that time. When Miss R. has been on L-DOPA for several weeks its advantages invariably become overweighed by its disadvantages, and she returns to a state of intense "block," crises, and tic-like impulsions. The form of her tics has varied a good deal on different occasions: in one of her periods on L-DOPA her crises were always accompanied by a palilalic verbigeration of the word "Honeybunch!" which she would repeat twenty or thirty times a minute for the entire day.

However deep and strange her pathological state, Miss R.

can invariably be "awakened" for a few seconds or minutes by external stimuli, although she is obviously quite unable to generate any such stimuli or calls-to-action for herself. If Miss A.—a fellow patient with dipsomania—drinks more than twenty times an hour at the water fountain, Miss R. cries, "Get away from that fountain, Margaret, or I'll clobber you!" or "Stop sucking that spout, Margaret, we all know what you really want to suck!" Whenever she hears my name being paged she yells out, "Dr. Sacks! Dr. Sacks!! They're after you again!" and continues to yell this until I have answered the page.

Miss R. is at her best when she is visited—as she frequently is—by any of her devoted family who fly in from all over the country to see her. At such time she is all agog with excitement, her blank masked face cracks into a smile, and she shows a great hunger for family gossip, though no interest at all in political events or other current "news"; at such times she is able to say a certain amount quite intelligibly, and in particular shows her fondness for jokes and mildly salacious indiscretions. Seeing Miss R. at this time one realizes what a "normal" and charming and alive personality is imprisoned or suspended by her ridiculous disease.

On a number of occasions I have asked Miss R. about the strange "nostalgia" which she showed in July 1969, and how she experiences the world generally. She usually becomes distressed and "blocked" when I ask such questions, but on a few occasions she has given me enough information for me to perceive the almost incredible truth about her. She indicates that in her "nostalgic" state she *knew* perfectly well that it was 1969 and that she was sixty-four years old, but that she *felt* that it was 1926 and she was twenty-one; she adds that she can't really imagine what it's like being older than twenty-one, because she has never really experienced it. For most of the time, however, there is "nothing, absolutely nothing, no thoughts at all" in her head, as if she is forced to block off an intolerable and insoluble anachronism—the almost half-century gap between her age as felt and experienced (her *ontological* age) and her actual or *official* age. It seems, in retrospect, as if the L-DOPA must have "de-blocked" her for a few days, and revealed to her a time-gap beyond comprehension or bearing, and that she has subsequently been forced to "re-block" herself and the possibility of any similar reaction to L-DOPA ever happening again. She continues to look much younger than her years; indeed, in a fundamental sense, she *is* much younger than her age. But she is a Sleeping Beauty whose "awakening" was unbearable to her, and who will never be awoken again.

# A DEAF WORLD

We are remarkably ignorant about deafness, which Dr. Johnson called "one of the most desperate of human calamities"—much more ignorant than an educated man would have been in 1886, or 1786. Ignorant and indifferent. During the last few months I have raised the subject with countless people and nearly always met with responses like: "Deafness? Don't know any deaf people. Never thought much about it. There's nothing *interesting* about deafness, is there?" This would have been my own response a few months ago.

Things changed for me when I was sent a fat book by Harlan Lane called *When the Mind Hears: A History of the Deaf,* which I opened with indifference, soon to be changed to astonishment, and then to something approaching

The text of this selection has been edited slightly from its original form in *Seeing Voices.*

incredulity. I discussed the subject with my friend and colleague Dr. Isabelle Rapin, who has worked closely with
the deaf for twenty-five years. I got to know better a
congenitally deaf colleague, a remarkable and highly gifted
woman, whom I had previously taken for granted.[1] I
started seeing, or exploring for the first time, a number of
deaf patients under my care. My reading rapidly spread
from Harlan Lane's history to *The Deaf Experience,* a collec-
tion of memoirs by and about the first literate deaf, edited
by Lane, and then to Nora Ellen Groce's *Everyone Here
Spoke Sign Language,* and to a great many other books. Now
I have an entire bookshelf on a subject that I had not
thought of even as existing six months ago, and have seen
some of the remarkable films that have been produced on
the subject.

One more acknowledgment by way of preamble. In

---

[1] This colleague, Lucy K., is so expert a speaker and lip-reader that I did not
realize at first that she was deaf. It was only when I chanced one day to turn my
head to one side as we were talking, inadvertently cutting off communication
instantly, that I realized she was not hearing me but lip-reading me ("lip-
reading" is an extremely inadequate word for the complex art of observation,
inference, and inspired guesswork which goes on). When the diagnosis of
deafness was made, at about twelve months, Lucy's parents had immediately
expressed their passionate desire that their daughter should speak and be a part
of the hearing world, and her mother devoted hours every day to an intensive
one-to-one tuition of speech—a grueling business that lasted twelve years. It
was only after this (at the age of fourteen) that Lucy learned Sign; it has always
been a second language, and one that does not come "naturally" to her. She
continued (with her excellent lip-reading and powerful hearing aids) in "normal" (hearing) classes in high school and college, and now works, with hearing
patients, at our hospital. She herself has mixed feeling about her status: "I
sometimes feel," she once said, "that I am between two worlds, that I don't
quite fit into either."

1969 W. H. Auden gave me a copy, his own copy, of *Deafness,* a remarkable autobiographical memoir by the South African poet and novelist David Wright, who became deaf at the age of seven. "You'll find it fascinating," he said. "It's a wonderful book." It was dotted with his own annotations (though I do not know whether he ever reviewed it). I skimmed it, without paying more attention, in 1969. But now I was to rediscover it for myself. David Wright is a writer who writes from the depths of his own experience—and not as a historian or scholar writes about a subject. Moreover, he is not alien to us. We can easily imagine, more or less, what it would be like to be him (whereas we cannot without difficulty imagine what it would be like to be someone born deaf, like the famous deaf teacher Laurent Clerc). Thus he can serve as a bridge for us, conveying us through his own experiences into the realm of the unimaginable. Since Wright is easier to read than the great mutes of the eighteenth century, he should if possible be read first—for he prepares us for them. Toward the close of the book he writes:

> Not much has been written about deafness by the deaf. Even so, considering that I did not become deaf till *after* I had learned the language, I am no better placed than a hearing person to imagine what it is like to be born into silence and reach the age of reason without acquiring a vehicle for thought and communication. Merely to try gives weight to the tremendous opening of St. John's

Gospel: In the beginning was the Word. How does one formulate concepts in such a condition?

It is this—the relation of language to thought—that forms the deepest, the ultimate issue when we consider what faces or may face those who are born, or very early become, deaf.

The term "deaf" is vague, or rather, is so general that it impedes consideration of the vastly differing degrees of deafness, degrees that are of qualitative, and even of "existential," significance. There are the "hard of hearing," fifteen million or so in the U.S. population, who can manage to hear some speech using hearing aids and a certain amount of care and patience on the part of those who speak to them. Many of us have parents or grandparents in this category—a century ago they would have used ear trumpets; now they use hearing aids.

There are also the "severely deaf," many as a result of ear disease or injury in early life; but with them, as with the hard of hearing, the hearing of speech is still possible, especially with the new, highly sophisticated, computerized, and "personalized" hearing aids now becoming available. Then there are the "profoundly deaf"—sometimes called "stone deaf"—who have no hope at all of hearing any speech, whatever imaginable technological advances are made. Profoundly deaf people cannot converse in the usual way—they must either lip-read (as David Wright did), or use sign language, or both.

It is not merely the degree of deafness that matters but—crucially—the age, or stage, at which it occurs. David Wright, in the passage already quoted, observes that he lost his hearing only after he had acquired language, and (this being the case) he cannot even imagine what it must be like for those who lack or have lost hearing before the acquisition of language. He brings this out in other passages.

> My becoming deaf when I did—if deafness had to be my destiny—was remarkably lucky. By the age of seven a child will have grasped the essentials of language, as I had. Having learned naturally how to speak was another advantage—pronunciation, syntax, inflexion, idiom, all had come by ear. I had the basis of a vocabulary which could easily be extended by reading. *All of these would have been denied me had I been born deaf or lost my hearing earlier than I did.* [Italics added.]

Wright speaks of the "phantasmal voices" that he hears when anyone speaks to him provided he can *see* the movement of their lips and faces, and of how he would "hear" the soughing of the wind whenever he saw trees or branches being stirred by the wind.[2] He gives a fascinating

[2]Wright uses Wordsworth's phrase, "eye-music," for such experiences, even when there is no accompanying auditory phantasm, and this is used by several deaf writers as a metaphor for their sense of visual patterns and beauty. It is

description of this first happening—of its *immediate* occurrence with the onset of deafness:

> [My deafness] was made more difficult to perceive because from the very first my eyes had unconsciously begun to translate motion into sound. My mother spent most of the day beside me and I understood everything she said. Why not? Without knowing it I had been reading her mouth all my life. When she spoke I seemed to hear her voice. It was an illusion which persisted even after I knew it was an illusion. My father, my cousin, everyone I had known, retained phantasmal voices. That they were imaginary, the projections of habit and memory, did not come home to me until I had left the hospital. One day I was talking with my cousin and he, in a moment of inspiration, covered his mouth with his hand as he spoke. Silence! Once and for all I understood that when I could not see I could not hear.[3]

Though Wright knows the sounds he "hears" to be "illusory"—"projections of habit and memory"—they remain

---

especially used of the recurrent motifs (the "rhymes," the "consonances," etc.) of Sign poetry.

[3] There is, of course, a "consensus" of the senses—objects are heard, seen, felt, smelt, all at once, simultaneously; their sound, sight, smell, feel all go together. This correspondence is established by experience and association. This is not, normally, something we are conscious of, although we would be very startled if something didn't sound like it looked—if one of our senses gave a discrepant impression. But we may be *made* conscious, very suddenly and startlingly, of the senses' correspondence, if we are suddenly deprived of a sense, or gain one.

intensely vivid for him throughout the decades of his deafness. For Wright, for those deafened after hearing is well established, the world may remain full of sounds even though they are "phantasmal."[4]

It is another matter entirely, and one that is essentially unimaginable, by the normal (and even by the postlingually deafened, like David Wright), if hearing is absent at birth, or lost in infancy before the language is acquired. Those so afflicted—the prelingually deaf—are in a category qualitatively different from all others. For these people, who have never heard, who have no possible auditory memories, images, or associations, there can never be even the illusion of sound. They live in a world of utter, unbroken soundlessness and silence.[5] These, the congenitally

[4] This hearing (that is, imagining) of "phantasmal voices," when lips are read, is quite characteristic of the *postlingually* deaf, for whom speech (and "inner speech") has once been an auditory experience. This is not "imagining" in the ordinary sense, but rather an instant and automatic "translation" of the visual experience into an auditory correlate (based on experience and association)—a translation that probably has a neurological basis (of experientially established visual-auditory connections). This does not occur, of course, in the *prelingually* deaf, who have no auditory experience or imagery to call upon. For them lipreading—as, indeed, ordinary reading—is an entirely visual experience; they see, but do not hear, the voice. It is difficult for us, as speaker-hearers, even to conceive such a visual "voice," as it is for those who have never heard to conceive an auditory voice.

The congenitally deaf, it should be added, may have the richest appreciation of (say) written English, of Shakespeare, even though it does not "speak" to them in an auditory way. It speaks to them, one must suppose, in an entirely visual way—they do not hear, they *see,* the "voice" of the words.

[5] This is the stereotypical view, and it is not altogether true. The congenitally deaf do not experience or complain of "silence" (any more than the blind experience or complain of "darkness"). These are our projections, or meta-

deaf, number perhaps a quarter of a million in this country. They make up a thousandth of the world's children.

It is with these and these only that we will be concerned here, for their situation and predicament are unique. Why should this be so? People tend, if they think of deafness at all, to think of it as less grave than blindness, to see it as a disadvantage, or a nuisance, or a handicap, but scarcely as devastating in a radical sense.

Whether deafness is "preferable" to blindness, if acquired in later life, is arguable; but to be born deaf is infinitely more serious than to be born blind—at least potentially so. For the prelingually deaf, unable to hear their parents, risk being severely retarded, if not permanently defective, in their grasp of language unless early and effective measures are taken. And to be defective in language, for a human being, is one of the most desperate of calamities, for it is only through language that we enter fully into our human estate and culture, communicate freely with our fellows, acquire and share information. If we cannot do this, we will be bizarrely disabled and cut off—whatever our desires, or endeavors, or native capacities. And indeed, we may be so little able to realize our intellectual capacities as to appear mentally defective.

---

phors, for their state. Moreover, those with the profoundest deafness may hear noise of various sorts and may be highly sensitive to vibrations of all kinds. This sensitivity to vibration can become a sort of accessory sense: thus Lucy K., although profoundly deaf, can immediately judge a chord as a "fifth" by placing a hand on the piano and can interpret voices on highly amplified telephones; in both cases what she seems to perceive are vibrations, not sounds.

It was for this reason that the congenitally deaf, or "deaf and dumb," were considered "dumb" (stupid) for thousands of years and were regarded by an unenlightened law as "incompetent"—to inherit property, to marry, to receive education, to have adequately challenging work—and were denied fundamental human rights. This situation did not begin to be remedied until the middle of the eighteenth century, when (perhaps as part of a more general enlightenment, perhaps as a specific act of empathy and genius) the perception and situation of the deaf were radically altered.

The *philosophes* of the time were clearly fascinated by the extraordinary issues and problems posed by a seemingly languageless human being. Indeed, the Wild Boy of Aveyron, when brought to Paris in 1800, was admitted to the National Institution for Deaf-Mutes, which was at the time supervised by the Abbé Roch-Ambroise Sicard, a founding member of the Society of Observers of Man, and a notable authority on the education of the deaf. As Jonathan Miller writes:

> As far as the members of this society were concerned the "savage" child represented an ideal case with which to investigate the foundations of human nature. . . . By studying a creature of this sort, just as they had previously studied savages and primitives, Red Indians and orangutans, the intellectuals of the late eighteenth century hoped to decide what was characteristic of Man. Perhaps it would now be possible to weigh the native endowment of the

human species and to settle once and for all the part that was played by society in the development of language, intelligence, and morality.

Here, of course, the two enterprises diverged, one ending in triumph, the other in complete failure. The Wild Boy never acquired language, for whatever reason or reasons. One insufficiently considered possibility is that he was, strangely, never exposed to sign language, but continually (and vainly) forced to try to speak. But when the "deaf and dumb" were properly approached, i.e., through sign language, they proved eminently educable, and they rapidly showed an astonished world how fully they could enter into its culture and life. This wonderful circumstance—how a despised or neglected minority, practically denied human status up to this point, emerged suddenly and startlingly upon the world stage (and the later tragic undermining of all this in the following century)—constitutes the opening chapter of the history of the deaf.

But let us, before launching on this strange history, go back to the wholly personal and "innocent" observations of David Wright ("innocent" because, as he himself stresses, he made a point of avoiding any reading on the subject until he had written his own book). At the age of eight, when it became clear that his deafness was incurable, and that without special measures his speech would regress, he was sent to a special school in England, one of the ruthlessly dedicated, but misconceived, rigorously "oral" schools, which are concerned above all to make the deaf speak like other children, and which have done so much harm to the prelingually deaf since their inception. The young David Wright was flabbergasted at his first encounter with the prelingually deaf.

Sometimes I took lessons with Vanessa. She was the first deaf child I had met. . . . But even to an eight-year-old like myself her general knowledge seemed strangely limited. I remember a geography lesson we were doing together, when Miss Neville asked,

"Who is the king of England?"

Vanessa didn't know; troubled, she tried to read sideways the geography book, which lay open at the chapter about Great Britain that we had prepared.

"King—king," began Vanessa.

"Go on," commanded Miss Neville.

"I know," I said.

"Be quiet."

"United Kingdom," said Vanessa.

I laughed.

"You are very silly," said Miss Neville. "How can a king be called 'United Kingdom'?"

"King United Kingdom," tried poor Vanessa, scarlet.

"Tell her if you know, [David]."

"King George the Fifth," I said proudly.

"It's not fair! It wasn't in the book!"

Vanessa was quite right of course; the chapter on the

geography of Great Britain did not concern itself with its political setup. She was far from stupid; but having been born deaf her slowly and painfully acquired vocabulary was still too small to allow her to read for amusement or pleasure. As a consequence there were almost no means by which she could pick up the fund of miscellaneous and temporarily useless information other children unconsciously acquire from conversation or random reading. Almost everything she knew she had been taught or made to learn. And this is a fundamental difference between hearing and deaf-born children—or was, in that pre-electronic era.

Vanessa's situation, one sees, was a serious one, despite her native ability; and it was helped only with much difficulty, if not actually perpetuated, by the sort of teaching and communication forced upon her. For in this progressive school, as it was regarded, there was an almost insanely fierce, righteous prohibition of sign language—not only of the standard British Sign Language but of the "sign-argot"— the rough sign language developed on their own by the deaf children in the school. And yet—this is also well described by Wright—signing flourished at the school, was irrepressible despite punishment and prohibition. This was young David Wright's first vision of the boys:

> Confusion stuns the eye, arms whirl like windmills in a hurricane . . . the emphatic silent vocabulary of the body— look, expression, bearing, glance of eye; hands perform their pantomime. Absolutely engrossing pandemonium. . . .

I begin to sort out what's going on. The seemingly cory-
bantic brandishing of hands and arms reduces itself to a
convention, a code which as yet conveys nothing. It is in
fact a kind of vernacular. The school has evolved its own
peculiar language or argot, though not a verbal one. . . .
All communications were supposed to be oral. Our own
sign-argot was of course prohibited. . . . But these rules
could not be enforced without the presence of the staff.
What I have been describing is not how we talked, but
how we talked among ourselves when no hearing person
was present. At such times our behaviour and conversation
were quite different. We relaxed inhibitions, wore no masks.

Such was the Northampton School in the English Mid-
lands, when David Wright went there as a pupil in 1927.
For him, as a postlingually deaf child, with a firm grasp of
language, the school was, manifestly, excellent. For Vanessa,
for other prelingually deaf children, such a school, with its
ruthlessly oral approach, was not short of a disaster. But a
century earlier, say, in the American Asylum for the Deaf,
opened a decade before in Hartford, Connecticut, where
there was free use of sign language between all pupils and
teachers, Vanessa would not have found herself pitifully
handicapped; she might have become a literate, perhaps
even literary, young woman of the sort who emerged and
wrote books during the 1830s.

————

The situation of the prelingually deaf, prior to 1750, was indeed a calamity: unable to acquire speech, hence "dumb" or "mute"; unable to enjoy free communication with even their parents and families; confined to a few rudimentary signs and gestures; cut off, except in large cities, even from the community of their own kind; deprived of literacy and education, all knowledge of the world; forced to do the most menial work; living alone, often close to destitution; treated by the law and society as little better than imbeciles—the lot of the deaf was manifestly dreadful.[6]

But what was manifest was as nothing to the destitution inside—the destitution of knowledge and thought that prelingual deafness could bring, in the absence of any communication or remedial measures. The deplorable state of the deaf aroused both the curiosity and the compassion of the *philosophes.* Thus the Abbé Sicard asked:

*Why* is the uneducated deaf person isolated in nature and unable to communicate with other men? *Why* is he reduced to this state of imbecility? Does his biological constitution differ from ours? Does he not have everything he needs for having sensations, acquiring ideas, and combining them to do everything that we do? Does he not get

[6] As early as the sixteenth century some of the deaf children of noble families had been taught to speak and read, through many years of tutoring, so that they could be recognized as persons under the law (mutes were not recognized) and could inherit their families' titles and fortunes. But before 1750, for the generality, for 99.9 percent of those born deaf, there was no hope of literacy or education.

sensory impressions from objects as we do? Are these not, as with us, the occasion of the mind's sensations and its acquired ideas? *Why* then does the deaf person remain stupid while we become intelligent?

To ask this question—never really or clearly asked before—is to grasp its answer, to see that the answer lies in the use of symbols. It is, Sicard continues, because the deaf person has "no symbols for fixing and combining ideas . . . that there is a total communication-gap between him and other people." But what was all-important, and had been a source of fundamental confusion since Aristotle's pronouncements on the matter, was the enduring misconception that symbols had to be speech. Perhaps indeed this passionate misperception, or prejudice, went back to biblical days: the subhuman status of mutes was part of the Mosaic code, and it was reinforced by the biblical exaltation of the voice and ear as the one and true way in which man and God could speak ("In the beginning was the Word"). And yet, overborne by Mosaic and Aristotelian thunderings, some profound voices intimated that this need not be so. Thus Socrates' remark in the *Cratylus* of Plato, which so impressed the youthful Abbé de l'Epée:

> If we had neither voice nor tongue, and yet wished to manifest things to one another, should we not, like those which are at present mute, endeavour to signify our meaning by the hands, head, and other parts of the body?

Or the deep, yet obvious, insights of the physician-philosopher Cardan in the sixteenth century:

It is possible to place a deaf-mute in a position to hear by reading, and to speak by writing . . . for as different sounds are conventionally used to signify different things, so also may the various figures of objects and words. . . . Written characters and ideas may be connected without the intervention of actual sounds.

In the sixteenth century the notion that the understanding of ideas did not depend upon the hearing of words was revolutionary.[7]

But it is not (usually) the ideas of philosophers that change reality; nor, conversely, is it the practice of ordinary people. What changes history, what kindles revolutions, is the meeting of the two. A lofty mind—that of the Abbé de l'Epée—had to meet a humble usage—the indigenous sign language of the poor deaf who roamed Paris—in order to make possible a momentous transformation. If we ask why this meeting had not occurred before, it has something to do with the vocation of the Abbé, who could not bear to think of the souls of the deaf-mute living and dying unshriven, deprived of the Catechism, the Scriptures, the Word of God; and it is partly owing to his humility—that

[7] There have been, however, purely written languages, such as the scholarly language used for over a thousand years by the elite Chinese bureaucracy, which was never spoken and, indeed, never intended to be spoken.

he *listened* to the deaf—and partly to a philosophical and linguistic idea then very much in the air—that of universal language, like the *speceium* of which Leibniz dreamed.[8] Thus, de l'Epée approached sign language not with contempt but with awe.

> The universal language that your scholars have sought for in vain and of which they have despaired, is here; it is right before your eyes, it is the mimicry of the impoverished deaf. Because you do not know it, you hold it in contempt, yet it alone will provide you with the key to all languages.

That this was a misapprehension—for sign language is not a universal language in this grand sense, and Leibniz's noble dream was probably a chimera—did not matter, was even an advantage.[9] For what mattered was that the Abbé

[8] De l'Epée exactly echoes his contemporary Rousseau, as do all the eighteenth-century descriptions of Sign. Rousseau (in his *Discourse on the Origin of Inequality* and his *Essay on the Origin of Language*) conceives of a primordial or original human language, in which everything has its true and natural name; a language so concrete, so particular, that it can catch the essence, the "itness," of everything; so spontaneous that it expresses all emotion directly, and so transparent that it is incapable of any evasion or deception. Such a language would be without (and indeed would have no need for) logic, grammar, metaphor, or abstractions—it would be a language not mediate, a symbolic expression of thought and feeling, but, almost magically, an *im*mediate one.

[9] This notion that sign language is uniform and universal, and enables deaf people all over the world to communicate with one another instantly, is still quite widespread. It is quite untrue. There are hundreds of different signed languages that have arisen independently wherever there are significant numbers of deaf people in contact.

paid minute attention to his pupils, acquired their language (which had scarcely ever been done by the hearing before). And then, by associating signs with pictures and written words, he taught them to read; and with this, in one swoop, he opened to them the world's learning and culture. De l'Epée's system of "methodical" signs—a combination of their own Sign with signed French grammar—enabled deaf students to write down what was said to them through a signing interpreter, a method so successful that, for the first time, it enabled ordinary deaf pupils to read and write French, and thus acquire an education. His school, founded in 1755, was the first to achieve public support. He trained a multitude of teachers for the deaf, who, by the time of his death in 1789, had established twenty-one schools for the deaf in France and Europe. The future of de l'Epée's own school seemed uncertain during the turmoil of revolution, but by 1791 it had become the National Institution for Deaf-Mutes in Paris, headed by the brilliant grammarian Sicard. De l'Epée's own book, as revolutionary as Copernicus' in its own way, was first published in 1776.

De l'Epée's book, a classic, is available in many languages. But what have not been available, have been virtually unknown, are the equally important (and, in some ways, even more fascinating) original writings of the deaf—the first deaf-mutes ever able to write. Harlan Lane and Franklin Philip have done a great service in making these so readily available to us in *The Deaf Experience*. Especially moving and important are the 1779 "Observations" of Pierre

Desloges—the first book to be published by a deaf person—now available in English for the first time. Desloges
himself, deafened at an early age, and virtually without
speech, provides us first with a frightening description of
the world, or unworld, of the languageless.

> At the beginning of my infirmity, and for as long as I was
> living apart from other deaf people . . . I was unaware of
> sign language. I used only scattered, isolated, and uncon-
> nected signs. I did not know the art of combining them to
> form distinct pictures with which one can represent vari-
> ous ideas, transmit them to one's peers, and converse in
> logical discourse.

Thus Desloges, though obviously a highly gifted man,
could scarcely entertain "ideas," or engage in "logical discourse," *until* he had acquired sign language (which, as is
usual with the deaf, he learned from someone deaf, in his
case from an illiterate deaf-mute). Desloges, though highly
intelligent, was intellectually disabled until he learned
Sign—and, specifically, to use the word that the British
neurologist Hughlings-Jackson was to use a century later in
regard to the disabilities attendant on aphasia, he was unable
to "propositionize." It is worth clarifying this by quoting
Hughlings-Jackson's own words:

> We do not either speak or think in words or signs only, but
> in words or signs referring to one another in a particular
> manner. . . . Without a proper interrelation of its parts, a

verbal utterance would be a mere succession of names, a word-heap, embodying no proposition. . . . The unit of speech is a proposition. Loss of speech (aphasia) is, therefore, the loss of power to propositionize . . . not only loss of power to propositionize aloud (to talk), but to propositionize either internally or externally. . . . The speechless patient has lost speech, not only in the popular sense that he cannot speak aloud, but in the fullest sense. We speak not only to tell other people what we think, but to tell ourselves what we think. Speech is a part of thought.

This is why, earlier, I spoke of prelingual deafness as being potentially far more devastating than blindness. For it may dispose, unless this is averted, to a condition of being virtually without language—and of being unable to "propositionize"—which must be compared to aphasia, a condition in which thinking itself can become incoherent and stunted. The languageless deaf may indeed be *as if* imbecilic—and in a particularly cruel way, in that intelligence, though present and perhaps abundant, is locked up so long as the lack of language lasts. Thus the Abbé Sicard is right, as well as poetic, when he writes of the introduction of Sign as "opening up the doors of . . . intelligence for the first time."

Nothing is more wonderful, or more to be celebrated, than something that will unlock a person's capacities and allow him to grow and think, and no one praises or portrays this with such fervor or eloquence as these suddenly liberated mutes, such as Pierre Desloges:

The [sign] language we use among ourselves, being a faithful image of the object expressed, is singularly appropriate for making our ideas accurate and for extending our comprehension by getting us to form the habit of constant observation and analysis. This language is lively; it portrays sentiment, and develops the imagination. No other language is more appropriate for conveying strong and great emotions.

But even de l'Epée was unaware, or could not believe, that sign language was a complete language, capable of expressing not only every emotion but every proposition and enabling its users to discuss any topic, concrete or abstract, as economically and effectively and grammatically as speech.

This indeed has always been evident, if only implicitly, to all native signers, but has always been denied by the hearing and speaking, who, however well intentioned, regard signing as something rudimentary, primitive, pantomimic, a poor thing. De l'Epée had this delusion—and it remains an almost universal delusion of the hearing now. On the contrary, it must be understood that Sign is the equal of speech, lending itself equally to the rigorous and the poetic—to philosophical analysis or to making love—indeed, with an ease that is sometimes greater than that of speech. (Indeed, if learned as a primary language, Sign may be used and maintained by the hearing as a continuing and at times preferred alternative to speech.)

The philosopher Condillac, who at first had seen deaf people as "sentient statues" or "ambulatory machines" incapable of thought or any connected mental activity, coming incognito to de l'Epée's classes, become a convert, and provided the first philosophic endorsement of his method and of sign language:

> From the language of action de l'Epée has created a methodical, simple, and easy art with which he gives his pupils ideas of every kind, and, I daresay, ideas more precise than the ones usually acquired with the help of hearing. When as children we are reduced to judging the meaning of words from the circumstances in which we hear them, it often happens that we grasp the meaning only approximately, and we are satisfied with this approximation all our lives. It is different with the deaf taught by de l'Epée. He has only one means for giving them sensory ideas; it is to analyze and to get the pupil to analyze with him. So he leads them from sensory to abstract ideas; we can judge how advantageous de l'Epée's action language is over the speech sounds of our governesses and tutors.

From Condillac to the public at large, who also flocked to de l'Epée's and Sicard's demonstrations, there came an enormous and generous change of heart, a welcoming of the previously outcast into human society. This period—

which now seems a sort of golden period in deaf history—
saw the rapid establishment of deaf schools, usually
manned by deaf teachers, throughout the civilized world,
the emergence of the deaf from neglect and obscurity,
their emancipation and enfranchisement, and their rapid
appearance in positions of eminence and responsibility—
deaf writers, deaf engineers, deaf philosophers, deaf intel-
lectuals, previously inconceivable, were suddenly possible.

When Laurent Clerc (a pupil of Massieu, himself a pupil
of Sicard) came to the United States in 1816, he had an
immediate and extraordinary impact, for American teachers up to this point had never been exposed to, never even
imagined, a deaf-mute of impressive intelligence and education, had never imagined the possibilities dormant in the
deaf. With Thomas Gallaudet, Clerc set up the American
Asylum for the Deaf, in Hartford, in 1817. As Paris—
teachers, *philosophes,* and public-at-large—was moved,
amazed, "converted" by de l'Epée in the 1770s, so America was to be converted fifty years later.

The atmosphere at the Hartford Asylum, and at other
schools soon to be set up, was marked by the sort of enthusiasm and excitement only seen at the start of grand intellectual and humanitarian adventures. The prompt and
spectacular success of the Hartford Asylum soon led to the
opening of other schools wherever there was sufficient
density of population, and thus of deaf students. Virtually

all the teachers of the deaf (nearly all of whom were fluent signers and many of whom were deaf) went to Hartford. The French sign system imported by Clerc rapidly amalgamated with the indigenous sign languages here—the deaf generate sign language wherever there are communities of deaf people; it is for them the easiest and most natural mode of communication—to form a uniquely expressive and powerful hybrid, American Sign Language (ASL).[10] A special indigenous strength—presented convincingly by Nora Ellen Groce in her book, *Everyone Here Spoke Sign Language*—was the contribution of the Martha's Vineyard deaf to the development of ASL. A substantial minority of the population there suffered from a hereditary deafness, and most of the island had adopted an easy and powerful sign language. Virtually all the deaf of the Vineyard were sent to the Hartford Asylum in its formative years, where they contributed to the developing national language the unique strength of their own.

[10] We lack sufficient direct knowledge of the evolution of ASL, especially in its first fifty years, when a far-reaching "creolization" occurred, as French Sign Language became Americanized. There was already a wide gulf between French Sign and the new creole ASL by 1867—Clerc himself commented on this—and this has continued to grow in the past hundred and twenty years. Nonetheless, there are still significant similarities between the two languages—sufficient for an American signer to feel somewhat at home in Paris.

In contrast, American signers have great difficulty understanding British Sign Language, which has quite different origins. Indigenous sign dialects may be extremely different: thus prior to 1817, a deaf American traveling across the States would encounter sign dialects incomprehensibly different from his own; and standardization was so slow in England that until quite recently signers in adjacent villages might be mutually unintelligible.

One has, indeed, a strong sense of pollination, of people coming to and fro, bringing regional languages, with all their idiosyncrasies and strengths, to Hartford, and taking back an increasingly polished and generalized language. The rise of deaf literacy and deaf education was as spectacular in the United States as it had been in France, and it soon spread to other parts of the world.

Lane estimates that by 1869 there were 550 teachers of the deaf worldwide and that 41 percent of the teachers of the deaf in the United States were themselves deaf. In 1864 Congress passed a law authorizing the Columbia Institution for the Deaf and the Blind in Washington to become a national deaf-mute college, the first institution of higher learning specifically for the deaf. Its first principal was Edward Gallaudet—the son of Thomas Gallaudet, who had brought Clerc to the United States in 1816. Gallaudet College, as it was later rechristened (it is now Gallaudet University), is still the only liberal arts college for deaf students in the world—though there are now several programs and institutes for the deaf associated with technical colleges. (The most famous of these is at the Rochester Institute of Technology, where there are more than 1,500 deaf students forming the National Technical Institute for the Deaf.)

The great impetus of deaf education and liberation, which had swept France between 1770 and 1820, thus continued its triumphant course in the United States until 1870 (Clerc, immensely active to the end and personally charismatic, died in 1869). And then—and this is the turning point in the entire story—the tide turned, turned against the use of Sign by and for the deaf, so that within twenty years the work of a century was undone.

Indeed, what was happening with the deaf and Sign was part of a general (and if one wishes, "political") movement of the time: a trend to Victorian oppressiveness, and conformism, intolerance of minorities, and minority usages, of every kind—religious, linguistic, ethnic. Thus it was at this time that the "little nations" and "little languages" of the world (for example, Wales and Welsh) found themselves under pressure to assimilate or conform.

Specifically, there had been for two centuries a countercurrent of feeling, from teachers and parents of deaf children, that the goal of deaf education should be teaching the deaf how to speak. Already, a century earlier, de l'Epée had found himself in implicit if not explicit opposition to Pereire, the greatest "oralist" or "demutizer" of his time, who dedicated his life to teaching deaf people how to speak; this was a task, indeed, for which dedication was needed, for it required years of the most intensive and arduous training, with one teacher working with one pupil, to have any hope of success, whereas de l'Epée could educate pupils by the hundred. Now, in the 1870s, a current that had been growing for decades, fed, paradoxically, by the immense success of the deaf-mute asylums and their spectacular demonstrations of the educability of the deaf, erupted and attempted to eliminate the very instrument of success.

There were, indeed, real dilemmas, as there had always

been, and they exist to this day. What good, it was asked, was the use of signs without speech? Would this not restrict deaf people, in daily life, to intercourse with other deaf people? Should not speech (and lipreading) be taught instead, allowing a full integration of the deaf into the general population? Should not signing be proscribed, lest it interfere with speech?[11]

But there is the other side of the argument. If the teaching of speech is arduous and occupies dozens of hours a week, might not its advantages be offset by these thousands of hours taken away from general education? Might one not end up with a functional illiterate who has, at best, a poor imitation of speech? What is "better," integration or education? Might one have both, by combining both speech and Sign? Or will any such attempted combination bring about, not the best, but the worst, of both worlds?

These dilemmas, these debates, of the 1870s seem to have been gathering force beneath the surface throughout

---

[11] The old terms "deaf and dumb" and "deaf-mute" referred to a supposed inadequacy of those born deaf to speak. They are, of course, perfectly capable of speech—they have the same speech apparatus as anyone else; what they lack is the ability to hear their own speech, and thus to monitor its sound by ear. Their speech, therefore, may be abnormal in amplitude and tone, with many omitted consonants and other speech sounds, sometimes so much so as to be unintelligible. Since deaf people cannot monitor their speech by ear, they have to learn to monitor it by other senses—by vision, touch, vibration-sense, and kinesthesia. Moreover, the prelingually deaf have no auditory image, no *idea* what speech actually sounds like, no idea of a sound-meaning correspondence. What is essentially an auditory phenomenon must be grasped and controlled by nonauditory means. It is this which poses great difficulties, and which may require thousands of hours of individual tuition to achieve.

a century of achievement—an achievement that could be seen, and was seen, by many, as perverse, as conducive to isolation and a set-apart people.

Edward Gallaudet himself was an open-minded man who traveled extensively in Europe in the late 1860s, touring deaf schools in fourteen countries. He found that the majority used both sign language and speech, that the sign language schools did as well as the oral schools as far as articulating speech was concerned, but obtained superior results in general education. He felt that articulation skills, though highly desirable, could not be the basis of primary instruction—that this had to be achieved, and achieved early, by Sign.

Gallaudet was balanced, but others were not. There had been a rash of "reformers"—Samuel Gridley Howe and Horace Mann were egregious examples—who clamored for an overthrow of the "old-fashioned" sign language asylums and for the introduction of "progressive" oralist schools. The Clarke School for the Deaf in Northampton, Massachusetts, was the first of these, opened in 1867. (It was the model and inspiration of the Northampton School in England, founded by the Reverend Thomas Arnold the following year.) But the most important and powerful of these "oralist" figures was Alexander Graham Bell, who was at once heir to a family tradition of teaching elocution and correcting speech impediments (his father and grandfather were both eminent in this), tied into a strange family mix of deafness denied (both his mother and his wife were deaf, but never acknowledged this) and, of course, a technological genius in his own right. When Bell threw all the weight of his immense authority and prestige into the advocacy of oralism, the scales were, finally, overbalanced and tipped, and at the notorious International Congress of Educators of the Deaf held at Milan in 1880, where deaf teachers were themselves excluded from the vote, oralism won the day and the use of Sign in schools was "officially" proscribed. Deaf pupils were prohibited from using their own "natural" language, and thenceforth forced to learn, as best they might, the (for them) "unnatural" language of speech. And perhaps this was in keeping with the spirit of the age, its overweening sense of science as power, of commanding nature and never deferring to it.

One of the consequences of this was that hearing teachers, not deaf teachers, now had to teach deaf students. The proportion of deaf teachers for the deaf, which was close to 50 percent in 1850, fell to 25 percent by the turn of the century, and to 12 percent by 1960. More and more, English became the language of instruction for deaf students, taught by hearing teachers, fewer and fewer of whom knew any sign language at all—the situation depicted by David Wright, at his school in the 1920s.

None of this would have mattered had oralism worked. But the effect, unhappily, was the reverse of what was desired—an intolerable price was exacted for the acquisition of speech. Deaf students of the 1850s who had been to the Hartford Asylum, or other such schools, were highly literate and educated—fully the equal of their hearing counterparts. Today the reverse is true. Oralism and the suppression of Sign have resulted in a dramatic deterioration in the educational achievement of deaf children and in the literacy of the deaf generally.

These dismal facts are known to all teachers of the deaf, however they are to be interpreted. Hans Furth, a psychologist whose work is concerned with cognition of the deaf, states that the deaf do as well as the hearing on tasks that measure intelligence without the need for acquired information. He argues that the congenitally deaf suffer from "information deprivation." There are a number of reasons for this. First, they are less exposed to the "incidental" learning that takes place out of school—for example, to that buzz of conversation that is the background of ordinary life; to television, unless it is captioned, etc. Second, the content of deaf education is meager compared to that of hearing children: so much time is spent teaching deaf children speech—one must envisage between five and eight years of intensive tutoring—that there is little time for transmitting information, culture, complex skills, or anything else.

Yet the desire to have the deaf speak, the insistence that they speak—and from the first, the odd superstitions that have always clustered around the use of sign language, to say nothing of the enormous investment in oral schools, allowed this deplorable situation to develop, practically unnoticed except by deaf people, who themselves being unnoticed had little to say in the matter. And it was only during the 1960s that historians and psychologists, as well as parents and teachers of deaf children, started asking, "What has happened? What *is* happening?" It was only in the 1960s and early 1970s that this situation reached the publics, in the form of novels such as Joanne Greenberg's *In This Sign* and more recently the powerful play (and movie) *Children of a Lesser God* by Mark Medoff.[12]

There is the perception that something must be done. But what? Typically, there is the seduction of compromise—that a "combined" system, combining sign and speech, will allow the deaf to become adept at both. A further compromise, containing a deep confusion, is suggested: having a language intermediate between English and Sign (i.e., a signed English). This category of confusion goes back a long way—back to de l'Epée's "Methodical Signs," which were an attempt to intermediate between French and Sign. But true sign languages are in fact complete in themselves: their syntax, grammar, and semantics are complete, but they have a different character from that of any spoken or written language. Thus it is not possible to transliterate a spoken tongue into Sign word by word or

---

[12] There had, of course, been other novels, like Carson McCullers's *The Heart Is a Lonely Hunter.* The figure of Mr. Singer, an isolated deaf man in a hearing world, in this book is quite different from the protagonists of Greenberg's novel, who are vividly conscious of their deaf identities. A huge social change, a change in social outlook, has occurred in the intervening thirty years, with above all, the emergence of a new self-consciousness.

phrase by phrase—their structures are essentially different. It is often imagined, vaguely, that sign language *is* English or French. It is nothing of the sort; it is itself, Sign. Thus, the "Signed English" now favored as a compromise is unnecessary, for no intermediary pseudo-language is needed. And yet, deaf people are forced to learn the signs not for the ideas and actions they want to express, but for phonetic English sounds they cannot hear.

Even now the use of signed English, in one form or another, is still favored against the use of ASL. Most teaching of the deaf, if done by signs, is done by signed English; most teachers of the deaf, if they know any sign, know this and not ASL; and the little cameos that appear on television screens all use signed English, not ASL. Thus, a century after the Milan conference, deaf people are still largely deprived of their own, indigenous language.

But what, more importantly, of the combined system by which students not only learn sign language but learn to lip-read and speak as well? Perhaps this is workable, if education takes account of which capacities are best developed at different phases of growth. The essential point is this: that profoundly deaf people show no native disposition whatever to speak. Speaking is an ability that must be taught them and is a labor of years. On the other hand, they show an immediate and powerful disposition to Sign, which as a visual language, is completely accessible to them. This is more apparent in the deaf children of deaf parents using Sign, who make their first signs when they are about six months old and have considerable sign fluency by the age of fifteen months.[13]

Language must be introduced and acquired as early as possible or its development may be permanently retarded and impaired, with all the problems in "propositionizing" which Hughlings-Jackson discussed. This can be done, with the profoundly deaf, only by Sign. Therefore deafness must be diagnosed as early as possible. Deaf children must first be exposed to fluent signers, whether these be their parents, or teachers, or whoever. Once signing is learned—and it may be fluent by three years of age—then all else may follow: a free intercourse of minds, a free flow of information, the acquisition of reading and writing, and perhaps that of speech. There is no evidence that signing inhibits the acquisition of speech. Indeed the reverse is probably so.

Have the deaf always and everywhere been seen as "handicapped" or "inferior"? Have they always suffered, must they always suffer, segregation and isolation? Can one imagine their situation otherwise? If only there were a

[13] Though there may be early development of a vocabulary of signs, the development of Sign grammar takes place at the same age, and in the same way, as the acquisition of speech grammar. Linguistic development thus occurs at the same rate in all children, deaf or hearing. If signs appear earlier than speech, it is because they are easier to make, for they involve relatively simple and slow movements of muscles, whereas speech involves the lightning coordination of hundreds of different structures, and only becomes possible in the second year of life. Yet it is intriguing that a deaf child at four months may make the sign for "milk," where a hearing child can only cry or look around. Perhaps all babies would be better off knowing a few signs!

world where being deaf did not matter, and in which all deaf people could enjoy complete fulfillment and integration! A world in which they would not even be perceived as "handicapped" or "deaf."[14]

Such worlds do exist, and have existed in the past, and such a world is portrayed in Nora Ellen Groce's beautiful and fascinating *Everyone Here Spoke Sign Language: Hereditary Deafness on Martha's Vineyard*. Through a mutation, a recessive gene brought out by inbreeding, a form of hereditary deafness existed for 250 years on Martha's Vineyard, Massachusetts, following the arrival of the first deaf settlers in the 1690s. By the mid-nineteenth century, scarcely an up-Island family was unaffected, and in some villages (Chilmark, West Tisbury) the incidence of deafness had risen to one in four. In response to this, the entire community

---

[14]Sicard imagined such a community:

> Could there not be in some corner of the world a whole society of deaf people? Well then! Would we think that these individuals were inferior, that they were unintelligent and lacked communication? They would certainly have a sign language, perhaps a language even richer than ours. This language would at least be unambiguous, always giving an accurate picture of the mind's affections. So why would this people be uncivilized? Why wouldn't they in fact have laws, government, police less mistrustful than our own?

The deaf themselves have had occasional impulses to deaf separatism or deaf "Zionism." In 1831 Edmund Booth suggested the formation of a deaf township or community, and in 1856 John James Flournoy the establishment of a deaf state, "out west." And in fantasy the idea is still active. Thus Lyson C. Sulla, the deaf hero of *Islay*, dreams of becoming governor of the state of Islay and making it a state "of, by, and for" deaf people.

learned Sign, and there was free and complete intercourse between the hearing and the deaf. Indeed the deaf were scarcely seen as "deaf," and certainly not seen as being at all "handicapped."[15]

In the astonishing interviews recorded by Groce, the island's older residents would talk at length, vividly and affectionately, about their former relatives, neighbors, and friends, usually without even mentioning that they were deaf. And it would only be if this question was specifically asked that there would be a pause and then, "Now you come to mention it, yes, Ebenezer *was* deaf and dumb." But Ebenezer's deaf-and-dumbness had never set him apart, and scarcely even been noticed as such: he had been seen, he was remembered, simply as "Ebenezer"—friend, neighbor, dory fisherman—not as some special, handicapped, set-apart

---

[15] There have been and are other isolated communities with a high incidence of deafness and unusually benign social attitudes to the deaf and their language.

There is an isolated village in the Yucatán where thirteen adults, and one baby, out of a population of about four hundred, are congenitally deaf—here again the whole village uses Sign. There are other deaf relatives—cousins, second cousins, etc.—in nearby villages.

The Sign they use is not "home sign," but a Mayan Sign that is clearly of some antiquity, because it is intelligible to all of these deaf people, even though they are scattered over hundreds of square miles, and have virtually no contact with each other. This is quite different from the Central Mexican Sign used in Merida and other cities—indeed, they are mutually unintelligible. The well-integrated, full lives of the rural deaf—in communities that accept them wholly, and have adapted by themselves learning Sign—is in great contrast to the low social, informational, educational, and linguistic level of the "city" deaf in Merida, who find themselves fit (after years of inadequate schooling) only for peddling or perhaps riding bike-taxis. One sees here how well the community often works, while the "system" does badly.

deaf-mute. The deaf on Martha's Vineyard loved, married, earned their livings, worked, thought, wrote as everyone else did—there were not set apart in any way, unless it was that they were, on the whole, better educated than their neighbors, for virtually all of the deaf on Martha's Vineyard were sent to be educated at the Hartford Asylum—and were often looked at as the most sagacious in the community.[16]

Intriguingly, even after the last deaf Islander had died in 1952, the hearing tended to preserve Sign among themselves, not merely for special occasions (telling dirty jokes, talking in church, communicating between boats, etc.) but generally. They would slip into it, involuntarily, sometimes in the middle of a sentence, because Sign is "natural" to all who learn it (as a primary language), and has an intrinsic beauty and excellence sometimes superior to speech.

I was so moved by Groce's book that the moment I finished it I jumped in the car, with only a toothbrush, a tape

[16] Besides its exemplary school for the deaf, the town of Fremont, California, offers unrivaled work opportunities for deaf people, as well as a rare degree of public and civic awareness and respect. The existence of thousands of deaf people in one area of Fremont has given rise to a fascinating bilingual and bicultural situation, whereby speech and Sign are used equally. In certain parts of town, one may see cafés where half the customers speak and half sign, Y's where deaf and hearing work out together, and athletic matches where deaf and hearing play together. There is here not only an interface—and a friendly one, between deaf and hearing—but a considerable fusion or diffusion of the two cultures, so that numbers of the hearing (especially children) have started to acquire Sign, usually quite unconsciously, by picking it up rather than deliberately learning it. Thus even here, in a bustling industrial Silicon Valley town in the 1980s (and there is a somewhat similar situation in Rochester, New York, where several thousand deaf students, some with deaf families, attend the NTID), we see that the benign Martha's Vineyard situation can reemerge.

recorder, and a camera—I had to see this enchanted island for myself. I saw how some of the oldest inhabitants still preserved Sign, delighted in it, among themselves. My first sight of this, indeed, was quite unforgettable. I drove up to the old general store in West Tisbury on a Sunday morning and saw half a dozen old people gossiping together on the porch. They could have been any old folks, old neighbors, talking together—until suddenly, very startlingly, they all dropped into Sign. They signed for a minute, laughed, then dropped back into speech. At this moment I knew I had come to the right place. And, speaking to one of the very oldest there, I found one other thing, of very great interest. This old lady, in her nineties, but sharp as a pin, would sometimes fall into a peaceful reverie. As she did so, she might have seemed to be knitting, her hands in constant complex motion. But her daughter, also a signer, told me she was not knitting but thinking to herself, thinking in Sign. And even in sleep, I was further informed, the old lady might sketch fragmentary signs on the counterpane— she was dreaming in Sign. Such phenomena cannot be accounted as merely social. It is evident that if a person has learned Sign as a primary language, his brain/mind will retain this, and use it, for the rest of that person's life, even though hearing and speech are freely available and unimpaired. Sign, I was now convinced, was a fundamental language of the brain.

# A SURGEON'S LIFE

Tourette's syndrome is seen in every race, every culture, every stratum of society; it can be recognized at a glance once one is attuned to it; and cases of barking and twitching, of grimacing, of strange gesturing, of involuntary cursing and blaspheming, were recorded by Aretaeus of Cappadocia almost two thousand years ago. Yet it was not clinically delineated until 1885, when George Gilles de la Tourette, a young French neurologist—a pupil of Charcot's and a friend of Freud's—put together these historical accounts with observations of some of his own patients. The syndrome as he described it was characterized, above all, by convulsive tics, by involuntary mimicry or repetition of others' words or actions (echolalia and echopraxia), and by the involuntary or compulsive utterances of curses and obscenities (coprolalia). Some individuals (despite their affliction) showed an odd insouciance or nonchalance; some a tendency to make strange, often witty, occasionally dream-like associations; some extreme impulsiveness and provoca-tiveness, a constant testing of physical and social boundaries; some a constant, restless reacting to the environment, a lunging at and sniffing of everything or a sudden flinging of objects; and yet others an extreme stereotypy and obses-siveness—no two patients were ever quite the same.

Any disease introduces a doubleness into life—an "it," with its own needs, demands, limitations. With Tourette's, the "it" takes the form of explicit compulsion, a multitude of explicit impulsions and compulsions: one is driven to do this, to do that, against one's own will, or in deference to the alien will of the "it." There may be a conflict, a com-promise, a collusion between these wills. Thus being "pos-sessed" can be more than a figure of speech for someone with an impulse disorder like Tourette's, and no doubt in the Middle Ages it was sometimes literally seen as "posses-sion." (Tourette himself was fascinated by the phenome-non of possession and wrote a play about the epidemic of demonic possession in medieval Loudun.)

But the relation of disease and self, "it" and "I," can be particularly complex in Tourette's, especially if it has been present from early childhood, growing up with the self, intertwining itself in every possible way. The Tourette's and the self shape themselves each to the other, come more and more to complement each other, until finally, like a long-married couple, they become a single, com-pound being. This relation is often destructive, but it can also be constructive, can add speed and spontaneity and a capacity for unusual and sometimes startling performance. For all its intrusiveness, Tourette's may be used creatively, too.

Yet in the years after its delineation, Tourette's tended to be seen not as an organic but as a "moral" disease—an expression of mischievousness or weakness of the will, to be treated by rectifying the will. From the 1920s to the 1960s, it tended to be seen as a psychiatric disease, to be treated by psychoanalysis or psychotherapy; but this, on the whole, proved ineffective, too. Then, with the demonstration, in the early 1960s, that the drug haloperidol could dramatically suppress its symptoms, Tourette's was regarded (in a sudden reversal) as a chemical disease, the result of an imbalance of a neurotransmitter, dopamine, in the brain. But all these views are partial, and reductive, and fail to do justice to the full complexity of Tourette's. Neither a biological nor a psychological nor a moral-social viewpoint is adequate; we must see Tourette's not only simultaneously from all three perspectives, but from an inner perspective, an existential perspective, that of the affected person himself. Inner and outer narratives here, as everywhere, must fuse.

Many professions, one would think, would be closed to someone with elaborate tics and compulsions or strange, antic behaviors, but this does not seem to be the case. Tourette's affects perhaps one person in a thousand, and we find people with Tourette's—sometimes the most severe Tourette's—in virtually every walk of life. There are Tourettic writers, mathematicians, musicians, actors, disc jockeys, construction workers, social workers, mechanics, athletes. Some things, one might think, would be completely out of the question—above all, perhaps, the intricate, precise, and steady work of a surgeon. This would have been my own belief not so long ago. But now, improbably, I know *five* surgeons with Tourette's.[1]

I first met Dr. Carl Bennett at a scientific conference on Tourette's in Boston. His appearance was unexceptionable—he was fiftyish, of middle size, with a brownish beard and mustache containing a hint of grey, and was dressed soberly in a dark suit—until he suddenly lunged or reached for the ground or jumped or jerked. I was struck both by his bizarre tics and by his dignity and calm. When I expressed incredulity about his choice of profession, he invited me to visit and stay with him, where he lived and practiced, in the town of Branford, in British Columbia— to do rounds at the hospital with him, to scrub with him, to see him in action. Now, four months later, in early October, I found myself in a small plane approaching Branford, full of curiosity and mixed expectations. Dr. Bennett met me at the airport, greeted me—a strange greeting, half lunge, half tic, a gesture of welcome idiosyncratically Tourettized—grabbed my case, and led the way to his car in an

---

[1] A further four surfaced (one an ophthalmic surgeon) following the original publication of this piece. In addition to these Tourettic surgeons, I now know of three Tourettic internists, two Tourettic neurologists, but only one Tourettic psychiatrist.

odd rapid skipping walk, with a skip each fifth step and sudden reachings to the ground as if to pick something up.

The situation of Branford is almost idyllic, nestled as it is in the shadow of the Rockies, in southeast British Columbia with Banff and its mountains to the north, and Montana and Idaho to the south; it lies in a region of great gentleness and fertility but is ringed with mountains, glaciers, lakes. Bennett himself has a passion for geography and geology; a few years ago he took a year off from his surgical practice to study both at the University of Victoria. As he drove, he pointed out moraines, stratifications, and other formations, so that what had at first seemed to my eyes a mere pastoral landscape became charged with a sense of history and chthonic forces, of immense geological vistas. Such keen, fierce attention to every detail, such constant looking below the surface, such examination and analysis, are characteristic of the restless, questioning Tourettic mind. It is, so to speak, the other side of the obsessive and perseverative tendencies, its disposition to reiterate, to touch again and again.

And, indeed, whenever the stream of attention and interest was interrupted, Bennett's tics and iterations immediately reasserted themselves—in particular, obsessive touchings of his mustache and glasses. His mustache had constantly to be smoothed and checked for symmetry, his glasses had to be "balanced"—up and down, side to side, diagonally, in and out—with sudden, ticcy touchings of the fingers, until they too, were exactly "centered." There were also occasional reachings and lungings with his right arm; sudden, compulsive touchings of the windshield with both forefingers

("The touching has to be symmetrical," he commented); sudden repositionings of his knees, or the steering wheel ("I have to have the knees symmetrical in relation to the steering wheel. They have to be *exactly* centered"); and sudden, high-pitched vocalizations, in a voice completely unlike his own, they sounded like "Hi, Patty," "Hi, there," and, on a couple of occasions, "Hideous!" (Patty, I learned later, was a former girlfriend, her name now enshrined in a tic.)[2]

There was little hint of this repertoire until we reached town and got obstructed by traffic lights. The lights did not annoy Bennett—we were in no hurry—but they did break up the driving, the kinetic melody, the swift, smooth stream of action, with its power to integrate mind and brain. The transition was very sudden: one minute, all was smoothness and action; the next, all was broken-upness, pandemonium,

---

[2]Tics can have an ambiguous status, partway between meaningless jerks or noises and meaningful acts. Though the tendency to tic is innate in Tourette's, the particular *form* of tics often has a personal or historical origin. Thus a name, a sound, a visual image, a gesture, perhaps seen years before and forgotten, may first be unconsciously echoed or imitated and then preserved in the stereotypic form of a tic. Such tics are like hieroglyphic, petrified residues of the past and may indeed, with the passage of time, become so hieroglyphic, so abbreviated, as to become unintelligible (as "God be with you" was condensed, collapsed, after centuries, to the phonetically similar but meaningless "good-bye"). One such patient, whom I saw long ago, kept making an explosive, guttural, trisyllabic noise, which revealed itself, on analysis, as a very accelerated, crushed rendering of *"Verboten!"* in a convulsive parody of his father's constantly forbidding German voice.

A recent correspondent, a woman with Tourette's, after reading an earlier version of this piece, wrote that " 'enshrinement' . . . is the perfect word to describe the interplay between life and tics—the process by which the former gets incorporated into the latter. . . . It is almost as if the Tourettic body becomes an expressive archive—albeit jumbled—of one's life experience."

riot. When Bennett was driving smoothly, one had the feeling not that the Tourette's was in any way being suppressed but that the brain and the mind were in a quite different mode of action.

Another few minutes, and we had arrived at his house, a charming, idiosyncratic house with a wild garden, perched on a hill overlooking the town. Bennett's dogs, rather wolflike, with strange, pale eyes, barked, wagged their tails, bounded up to us as we drove in. As we got out of the car, he said "Hi, puppies!" in the same quick, odd, high, crushed voice he had earlier used for "Hi, Patty!" He patted their heads, a ticklike, convulsive patting, a quick-fire volley of five pats to each, delivered with a meticulous symmetry and synchrony. "They're grand dogs, half-Eskimo, half-malamute," he said. "I felt I should get two of them, so they could companion each other. They play together, sleep together, hunt together—everything." And, I thought, are patted together: Did he get two dogs partly because of his own symmetrical, symmetrizing compulsions? Now, hearing the dogs bark, his sons ran out—two handsome teenage kids. I had a sudden feeling that Bennett might cry "Hi, kiddies!" in his Touretty voice and pat their heads, too, in synchrony, symmetrically. But he introduced them, Mark and David, individually to me. And then, as we entered the house, he introduced me to his wife, Helen, who was preparing a late-afternoon tea for all of us.

As we sat at the table, Bennett was repeatedly distracted by tics—a compulsive touching of the glass lampshade above his head. He had to tap the glass gently with the nails of both forefingers, to produce a sharp, half-musical click or, on occasion, a short salvo of clicks. A third of his time was taken up with this ticcing and clicking, which he seemed unable to stop. Did he have to do it? Did he have to sit there?

"If it were out of reach, would you still have to click it?" I asked.

"No," he said. "It depends entirely on how I'm situated. It's all a question of space. Where I am now, for example, I have no impulse to reach over to that brick wall, but if I were in range I'd have to touch it perhaps a hundred times." I followed his glance to the wall and saw that it was pockmarked, like the moon, from his touchings and jab-bings, and, beyond it, the refrigerator door, dented and battered, as if from the impact of meteorites or projectiles. "Yeah," Bennett said, now following my glance. "I fling things—the iron, the rolling pin, the saucepan, whatever—I fling things at it if I suddenly get enraged." I digested this information in silence. It added a new dimension—a dis-quieting, violent one—to the picture I was building and seemed completely at odds with the genial, tranquil man before me.[3]

---

[3] Some people with Tourette's have flinging tics—sudden, seemingly motive-less urges or compulsions to throw objects—quite different from Bennett's flinging in rage. There may be a very brief premonition—enough, in one case, to yell a warning "Duck!"—before a dinner plate, a bottle of wine, or what-ever is flung convulsively across the room. Identical throwing tics occurred in some of my postencephalitic patients when they were overstimulated by L-DOPA. (I see somewhat similar flinging behaviors—though not tics—in my two-year-old godson, now in a stage of primal antinomianism and anarchy.)

"If the light so disturbs you, why do you sit near it?" I asked.

"Sure, it's 'disturbance,'" Bennett answered. "But it's also stimulation. I like the feeling and the sound of the click. But, yeah, it can be a great distraction. I can't study here, in the dining room—I have to go to my study, out of reach of the lamp."

The sense of personal space, of the self in relation to other objects and other people, tends to be markedly altered in Tourette's syndrome. I know many people with Tourette's who cannot tolerate sitting in a restaurant within touching distance of other people and may feel compelled, if they cannot avoid this, to reach out or lunge convulsively toward them. This intolerance may be especially great if the "provoking" person is behind the Touretter. Many people with Tourette's, therefore, prefer corners, where they are at a "safe" distance from others, and there is nobody behind them.[4] Analogous problems may arise, on occasion, when driving; there may be a sense that other vehicles are "too close" or "looming," even that they are suddenly "zooming," when they are (a non-Tourettic person would judge) at a normal distance. There may also be, paradoxically, a tendency to be "attracted" to other vehicles, to drift or

---

[4] This was comically shown on one occasion when I went to a restaurant for dinner with three Tourettic friends in Los Angeles. All three of them at once rushed for the corner seat—not, I think, in any competitive spirit, but because each saw it as an existential-neural necessity. The lucky one was able to sit calmly in his place, while the other two were constantly lunging at other diners behind them.

veer toward them—though the consciousness of this, and a greater speed of reaction, usually serves to avert any mishaps. (Similar illusions and urges, stemming from abnormalities in the neural basis of personal space, may occasionally be seen in parkinsonism, too.)

Another expression of Bennett's Tourette's—very different from the sudden impulsive or compulsive touching—is a slow, almost sensuous pressing of the foot to mark out a circle in the ground all around him. "It seems to me almost instinctual," he said when I asked him about it. "Like a dog marking its territory. I feel it in my bones. I think it is something primal, prehuman—maybe something that all of us, without knowing it, have in us. But Tourette's 'releases' these primitive behaviors."[5]

Bennett sometimes calls Tourette's "a disease of disinhibition." He says there are thoughts, not unusual in themselves, that anyone might have in passing but that are normally inhibited. With him, such thoughts perseverate in the back of the mind, obsessively, and burst out suddenly, without his consent or intention. Thus, he says, when the weather is nice he may want to be out in the sun getting a tan. This thought will be in the back of his mind while he is seeing his patients in the hospital and will

---

[5] Tourette's should not be regarded as a psychiatric disorder, but as a neurobiological disorder of a hyperphysiological sort, in which there may occur subcortical excitation and spontaneous stimulation of many phylogenetically primitive centers in the brain. A similar stimulation or release of "primitive" behaviors may be seen with the excitatory lesions of encephalitis lethargica, such as I describe in *Awakenings*. These were often apparent in the early days of the illness and became prominent again with the stimulation of L-DOPA.

emerge in sudden, involuntary utterances. "The nurse may say, 'Mr. Jones has abdominal pain,' and I'm looking out the window saying, 'Tanning rays, tanning rays.' It might come out five hundred times in a morning. People in the ward must hear it—they can't *not* hear it—but I guess they ignore it or feel that it doesn't matter."

Sometimes the Tourette's manifests itself in obsessive thoughts and anxieties. "If I'm worried about something," Bennett told me as we sat around the table, "say, I hear a story about a kid being hurt, I have to go up and tap the wall and say, 'I hope it won't happen to mine.'" I witnessed this for myself a couple of days later. There was a news report on TV about a lost child, which distressed and agitated him. He instantly began touching his glasses (top, bottom, left, right, top, bottom, left, right), centering and recentering them in a fury. He made "whoo, whoo" noises, like an owl, and muttered sotto voce, "David, David—is *he* all right?" Then he dashed from the room to make sure. There was an intense anxiety and overconcern; an immediate alarm at the mention of any lost or hurt child; an immediate identification with himself, with his own children; an immediate, superstitious need to check up.

After tea, Bennett and I went out for a walk, past a little orchard heavy with apples and on up the hill overlooking the town, the friendly malamutes gamboling around us. As we walked, he told me something of his life. He did not know whether anyone in his family had Tourette's—he was an adopted child. His own Tourette's had started when he was about seven. "As a kid, growing up in Toronto, I wore glasses, I had bands on my teeth, *and* I twitched," he said. "That was the coup de grâce. I kept my distance. I was a loner; I'd go for long hikes by myself. I never had friends phoning all the time, like Mark—the contrast is very great." But being a loner and taking long hikes by himself toughened him as well, made him resourceful, gave him a sense of independence and self-sufficiency. He was always good with his hands and loved the structure of natural things—the way rocks formed, the way plants grew, the way animals moved, the way muscles balanced and pulled against each other, the way the body was put together. He decided very early that he wanted to be a surgeon.

Anatomy came "naturally" to him, he said, but he found medical school extremely difficult, not merely because of his tics and touchings, which became more elaborate with the years, but because of strange difficulties and obsessions that obstructed the act of reading. "I'd have to read each line many times," he said. "I'd have to line up each paragraph to get all four corners symmetrically in my visual field." Besides this lining up of each paragraph, and sometimes of each line, he was beset by the need to "balance" syllables and words, by the need to "symmetrize" the punctuation in his mind, by the need to check the frequency of a given letter, and by the need to repeat words or phrases or lines to himself.[6] All this made it impossible to

[6]Such tendencies, common in Tourette's syndrome, are also seen in patients with post-encephalitic syndromes. Thus my patient Miriam H. had compul-

read easily and fluently. Those problems are still with him and make it difficult for him to skim quickly, to get the gist, or to enjoy fine writing or narrative or poetry. But they did force him to read painstakingly and to learn his medical texts very nearly by heart.

When he got out of medical school, he indulged his interest in faraway places, particularly the North: he worked as a general practitioner in the Northwest Territories and the Yukon and worked on icebreakers circling the Arctic. He had a gift for intimacy and grew close to the Eskimos he worked with and he became something of an expert in polar medicine. And when he married, in 1968—he was twenty-eight—he went with his bride around the world and gratified a boyhood wish to climb Kilimanjaro.

For the past seventeen years, he has practiced in small, isolated communities in western Canada—first, for twelve years as a general practitioner in a small city. Then, five years ago, when the need to have mountains, wild country, and lakes on his doorstep grew stronger, he moved to Branford. ("And here I will stay. I never want to leave it.") Branford, he told me, has the right "feel." The people are warm but not chummy, they keep a certain distance. There is a natural well-bredness and civility. The schools are of high quality, there is a community college, there are theaters and bookstores—Helen runs one of them—but there is also a strong feeling for the outdoors, for the wilds.

---

sions to count the number of *e*'s on every page she read; to say, or write, or spell sentences backward; to divide people's faces into juxtapositions of geometric figures, and to balance visually, to symmetrize, everything she saw.

There is much hunting and fishing, but Bennett prefers backpacking and climbing and cross-country skiing.

When Bennett first came to Branford, he was regarded, he thought, with a certain suspicion. "A surgeon who twitches! Who needs him? What next?" There were no patients at first, and he did not know if he could make it there, but gradually he won the town's affection and respect. His practice began to expand, and his colleagues, who had initially been startled and incredulous, soon came to trust and accept him, too, and to bring him fully into the medical community. "But enough said," he concluded as we returned to the house. It was almost dark now, and the lights of Branford were twinkling. "Come to the hospital tomorrow—we have a conference at seven-thirty. Then I'll do outpatients and rounds on my patients. And Friday I operate—you can scrub with me."

I slept soundly in the Bennetts' basement room that night, but in the morning I woke early, roused by a strange whirring noise in the room next to mine—the playroom. The playroom door had translucent glass panels. As I peered through them, still half-asleep, I saw what appeared to be a locomotive in motion—a large, whirring wheel going round and round and giving off puffs of smoke and occasional hoots. Bewildered, I opened the door and peeked in. Bennett, stripped to the waist, was pedaling furiously on an exercise bike while calmly smoking a large pipe. A pathology book was open before him—turned, I observed, to the chapter on neurofibromatosis. This is how he invariably begins each morning—a half hour on his bike, puffing his favorite pipe, with a pathology or surgery book open to the day's work before him. The pipe, the rhythmic exercise, calm him. There are no tics, no compulsions—at most, a little hooting. (He seems to imagine at such times that he is a prairie train.) He can read, thus calmed, without his usual obsessions and distractions.

But as soon as the rhythmic cycling stopped, a flurry of tics and compulsions took over; he kept digging at his belly, which was trim, and muttering, "Fat, fat, fat . . . fat, fat, fat . . . fat, fat, fat," and then, puzzlingly, "Fat and a quarter tit." (Sometimes the "tit" was left out.)

"What does it mean?" I asked.

"I have no idea. Nor do I know where 'Hideous' comes from—it suddenly appeared one day two years ago. It'll disappear one day, and there will be another word instead. When I'm tired, it turns into 'Gideous.' One cannot always find sense in these words; often it is just the sound that attracts me. Any odd sound, any odd name, may start repeating itself, get me going. I get hung up with a word for two or three months. Then, one morning, it's gone, and there's another one in its place." Knowing his appetite for strange words and sounds, Bennett's sons are constantly on the lookout for "odd" names—names that sound odd to an English-speaking ear, many of them foreign. They scan the papers and their books for such words, they listen to the radio and TV, and when they find a "juicy" name, they add it to a list they keep. Bennett says of this list, "It's about the most valuable thing in the house." He calls its words "candy for the mind."

This list was started six years ago, after the name Oginga Odinga, with its alliterations, got Bennett going—and now it contains more than two hundred names. Of these, twenty-two are "current"—apt to be regurgitated at any moment and chewed over, repeated, and savored internally. Of the twenty-two, the name of Slavek J. Hurka—an industrial-relations professor at the University of Saskatchewan, where Helen studied—goes the furthest back; it started to echolale itself in 1974 and has been doing so, without significant breaks, for the last seventeen years. Most words last only a few months. Some of the names (Boris Blank, Floyd Flake, Morris Gook, Lubor J. Zink) have a short, percussive quality. Others (Yelberton A. Tittle, Babaloo Mandel) are marked by euphonious polysyllabic alliterations. Echolalia freezes sounds, arrests time, preserves stimuli as "foreign bodies" or echoes in the mind, maintaining an alien existence, like implants. It is only the sound of the words, their "melody," as Bennett says, that implants them in his mind; their origins and meanings and associations are irrelevant. (There is a similarity here to his "enshrinement" of names as tics.)

"It is similar with the number compulsions," he said. "Now I have to do everything by threes or fives, but until a few months ago it was fours and sevens. Then one morning I woke up—*four* and *seven* had gone, but *three* and *five* had appeared instead. It's as if one circuit were turned on upstairs, and another turned off. It doesn't seem to have anything to do with *me*."

It is always the odd, the unusual, the salient, the carica-turable, that catch the ear and eye of the Touretter and tend to provoke elaboration and imitation.[7] This is well brought out in the personal account cited by Meige and Feindel in 1902:

I have always been conscious of a predilection for imita-tion. A curious gesture or bizarre attitude affected by any one was the immediate signal for an attempt on my part at its reproduction, and is still. Similarly with words or phrases, pronunciation or intonation, I was quick to mimic any peculiarity.

When I was thirteen years old I remember seeing a man with a droll grimace of eyes and mouth, and from that moment I gave myself no respite until I could imitate it accurately. . . . For several months I kept repeating the old gentleman's grimace involuntarily. I had, in short, begun to tic.

[7]The name of an eminent researcher on Tourette's syndrome—Dr. Abuzza-hab—has an almost diagnostic power, provoking grotesque, perseverative elab-orations in Tourette's (Abuzzahuzzahab, etc.). The power of the unusual to excite and impress is not, of course, confined to Touretters. The anonymous author of the ancient mnemotechnic text *Ad Herennium* described it, two thousand years ago, as a natural bent of the mind and one to be exploited for fixing images more firmly in the mind:

When we see in everyday life things that are petty, ordinary, and banal, we generally fail to remember them, because the mind is not being stirred by anything novel or marvellous. But if we see or hear something exceptionally base, dishonourable, unusual, great, unbeliev-able, or ridiculous, that we are likely to remember for a long time. . . . Ordinary things easily slip from the memory while the striking and the novel stay longer in the mind. . . . Let art, then, imitate nature.

At 7:25 we drove into town. It took barely five minutes to get to the hospital, but our arrival there was more complicated than usual, because Bennett had unwittingly become notorious. He had been interviewed by a magazine a few weeks earlier, and the article had just come out. Everyone was smiling and ribbing him about it. A little embarrassed, but also enjoying it, Bennett took the joking in good part. ("I'll never live it down—I'll be a marked man now.") In the doctors' common room, Bennett was clearly very much at ease with his colleagues, and they with him. One sign of this ease, paradoxically, was that he felt free to Tourette with them—to touch or tap them gently with his fingertips or, on two occasions when he was sharing a sofa, to suddenly twist on his side and tap his colleague's shoulder with his toes—a practice I had observed in other Touretters. Bennett is somewhat cautious with his Tourettisms on first acquaintance and conceals or downplays them until he gets to know people. When he first started working at the hospital, he told me, he would skip in the corridors only after checking to be sure that no one was looking; now when he skips or hops no one gives it a second glance.

The conversations in the common room were like those in any hospitals—doctors talking among themselves about unusual cases. Bennett himself, lying half-curled on the floor, kicking and thrusting one foot in the air, described an unusual case of neurofibromatosis—a young man whom he had recently operated on. His colleagues listened attentively. The abnormality of the behavior and the complete normality of the discourse formed an extraordinary contrast. There was something bizarre about the whole scene, but it was evidently so common as to be unremarkable and no longer attracted the slightest notice. But an outsider seeing it would have been stunned.

After coffee and muffins, we repaired to the surgical-outpatients department, where half a dozen patients awaited Bennett. The first was a trail guide from Banff, very western in plaid shirt, tight jeans, and cowboy hat. His horse had fallen and rolled on top of him, and he had developed an immense pseudocyst of the pancreas. Bennett spoke with the man—who said the swelling was diminishing—and gently, smoothly palpated the fluctuant mass in his abdomen. He checked the sonograms with the radiologist—they confirmed the cyst's recession—and then came back and reassured the patient. "It's going down by itself. It's shrinking nicely—you won't be needing surgery after all. You can get back to riding. I'll see you in a month." And the trail guide, delighted, walked off with a jaunty step. Later, I had a word with the radiologist. "Bennett's not only a whiz at diagnosis," he said. "He's the most compassionate surgeon I know."

The next patient was a heavy woman with a melanoma on her buttock, which needed to be excised at some depth. Bennett scrubbed up, donned sterile gloves. Something about the sterile field, the prohibition, seemed to stir his Tourette's; he made sudden darting motions, or incipient motions, of his sterile, gloved right hand toward the ungloved, unwashed, "dirty" part of his left arm. The patient eyed this without expression. What did she think, I wondered, of this odd darting motion, and the sudden convulsive shakings he also made with his hand? She could not have been entirely surprised, for her G.P. must have prepared her to some extent, must have said, "You need a small operation. I recommend Dr. Bennett—he's a wonderful surgeon. I have to tell you that he sometimes makes strange movements and sounds—he has a thing called Tourette's syndrome—but don't worry, it doesn't matter. It never affects his surgery."

Now, the preliminaries over, Bennett got down to the serious work, swabbing the buttock with an iodine antiseptic and then injecting local anesthetic, with an absolutely steady hand. But as soon as the rhythm of action was broken for a moment—he needed more local, and the nurse held out the vial for him to refill his syringe—there was once again the darting and near-touching. The nurse did not bat an eyelid; she had seen it before and knew he would not contaminate his gloves. Now, with a firm hand, Bennett made an oval incision an inch to either side of the melanoma, and in forty seconds he had removed it, along with a Brazil-nut-shaped wodge of fat and skin. "It's out!" he said. Then, very rapidly, with great dexterity, he sewed the margins of the wound together, putting five neat knots on each nylon stitch. The patient, twisting her head, watched him as he sewed and joshed him: "Do you do all the sewing at home?"

He laughed. "Yes. All except the socks. But no one darns socks these days."

She looked again. "You're making quite a quilt."

The whole operation completed in less than three minutes, Bennett cried, "Done! Here's what we took." He held the lump of flesh before her.

"Ugh!" she exclaimed, with a shudder. "Don't show me. But thanks anyway."

All this looked highly professional from beginning to end, and, apart from the dartings and near-touchings, non-Tourettic. But I couldn't decide about Bennett's showing the excised lump to the patient. ("Here!") One may show a gallstone to a patient, but does one show a bleeding, misshapen piece of fat and flesh? Clearly, she didn't want to see it, but Bennett wanted to show it, and I wondered if this urge was part of his Tourettic scrupulosity and exactitude, his need to have everything looked at and understood. I had the same thought later in the morning, when he was seeing an old lady in whose bile duct he had inserted a T-tube. He went to great lengths to draw the tube, to explain all the anatomy, and the old lady said, "I don't want to know it. Just do it!"

Was this Bennett the Touretter being compulsive or Professor Bennett the lecturer on anatomy? (He gives weekly anatomy lectures in Calgary.) Was it simply an expression of his meticulousness and concern? An imagining, perhaps, that all patients shared his curiosity and love of detail? Some patients doubtless did, but obviously not these.

So it went on through a lengthy outpatient list. Bennett is evidently a very popular surgeon, and he saw or operated on each patient swiftly and dexterously, with an absolute and single-minded concentration, so that when they saw him they knew they had his whole attention. They forgot that they had waited, or that there were others still waiting, and felt that for him they were the only people in the world.

Very pleasant, very real, the surgeon's life, I kept thinking—direct, friendly relationships, especially clear with outpatients like this. An immediacy of relation, of work, of results, of gratification—much greater than with a physician, especially a neurologist (like me). I thought of my mother, how much she enjoyed the surgeon's life, and how I always loved sitting in at her surgical-outpatient rounds. I could not become a surgeon myself, because of an incorrigible clumsiness, but even as a child I had loved the surgeon's life, and watching surgeons at work. This love, this pleasure, half-forgotten, came back to me with great force as I observed Bennett with his patients; made me want to be more than a spectator; made me want to do something, to hold a retractor, to join in the surgery somehow.

Bennett's last patient was a young mechanic with extensive neurofibromatosis, a bizarre and sometimes cancerous disease that can produce huge brownish swellings and protruding sheets of skin, disfiguring the whole body.[8] This young man had had a huge apron of tissue hanging down from his chest, so large that he could lift it up and cover his head, and so heavy that it bowed him forward with its weight. Bennett had removed this a couple of weeks ear-

---

[8] This was long presumed to have been the condition that afflicted the famous Elephant Man, John Merrick, although there is some suggestion that he may have had Proteus syndrome instead.

lier—a massive procedure—with great expertise, and was now examining another huge apron descending from the shoulders, and great flaps of brownish flesh in the groins and armpits. I was relieved that he did not tic "Hideous!" as he removed the stitches from the surgery, for I feared the impact of such a word being uttered aloud, even if it was nothing but a long-standing verbal tic. But, mercifully, there was no "Hideous!"; there were no verbal tics at all, until Bennett was examining the dorsal skin flap and let fly a brief "Hid—," the end of the word omitted by a tactful apocope. This, I learned later, was not a conscious suppression—Bennett had no memory of the tic—and yet it seemed to me there must have been, if not a conscious, then a subconscious solicitude and tact at work. "Fine young man," Bennett said, as we went outside. "Not self-conscious. Nice personality, outgoing. Most people with this would lock themselves in a closet." I could not help feeling that his words could also be applied to himself. There are many people with Tourette's who become agonized and self-conscious, withdraw from the world, and lock themselves in a closet. Not so Bennett: he had struggled against this; he had come through and braved life, braved people, braved the most improbable of professions. All his patients, I think, perceive this, and it is one of the reasons they trust him so.

The man with the skin flap was the last of the outpatients, but for Bennett, immensely busy, there was only a brief break before an equally long afternoon with his inpatients

on the ward. I excused myself from this to take an afternoon off and walk around the town. I wandered through
Branford with the oddest sense of déjà vu and jamais vu
mixed; I kept feeling that I had seen the town before, but
then again that it was new to me. And then, suddenly, I had
it—yes, I had seen it, I had been here before, had stopped
here for a night in August 1960, when I was hitchhiking
through the Rockies, to the West. It had a population then
of only a few thousand and consisted of little more than a
few dusty streets, motels, bars—a crossroads, little more
than a truck stop in the long trek across the West. Now its
population was twenty thousand, Main Street a gleaming
boulevard filled with shops and cars; there was a town hall,
a police station, a regional hospital, several schools—it was
this that surrounded me, the overwhelming present, yet
through it I saw the dusty crossroads and the bars, the
Branford of thirty years before, still strangely vivid, because
never updated, in my mind.

Friday is operating day for Bennett, and he was scheduled
to do a mastectomy. I was eager to join him, to see him in
action. Outpatients are one thing—one can always concentrate for a few minutes—but how would he conduct
himself in a lengthy and difficult procedure demanding
intense, unremitting concentration, not for seconds or minutes, but for hours?

Bennett preparing for the operating room was a startling
sight. "You should scrub next to him," his young assistant

said. "It's quite an experience." It was indeed, for what I saw in the outpatient clinic was magnified here: constant sudden dartings and reachings with the hands, almost but never quite touching his unscrubbed, unsterile shoulder, his assistant, the mirror; sudden lungings; and touchings of his colleagues with his feet; and a barrage of vocalizations—"Hooty-hooo! Hooty-hooo!"—suggestive of a huge owl.

The scrubbing over, Bennett and his assistant were gloved and gowned, and they moved to the patient, already anesthetized, on the table. They looked briefly at a mammogram on the X-ray box. Then Bennett took the knife, made a bold, clear incision—there was no hint of any ticcing or distraction—and moved straightaway into the rhythm of the operation. Twenty minutes passed, fifty, seventy, a hundred. The operation was often complex—vessels to be tied, nerves to be found—but the action was confident, smooth, moving forward at its own pace, with never the slightest hint of Tourette's. Finally, after two and a half hours of the most complex, taxing surgery, Bennett closed up, thanked everybody, yawned, and stretched. Here, then, was an entire operation without a trace of Tourette's. Not because it had been suppressed, or held in—there was never any sign of control or constraint—but because, simply, there was never any impulse to tic. "Most of the time when I'm operating, it never even crosses my mind that I have Tourette's," Bennett says. His whole identity at such times is that of a surgeon at work, and his entire psychic and neural organization becomes aligned with this, becomes active, focused, at ease, un-Tourettic. It is only if the operation is broken for a few minutes—to review a special X ray taken during the surgery, for example—that Bennett, waiting, unoccupied, remembers that he *is* Tourettic, and in that instant he becomes so. As soon as the flow of the operation resumes, the Tourette's, the Tourettic identity, vanishes once again. Bennett's assistants, though they have known him and worked with him for years, are still astounded whenever they see this. "It's like a miracle," one of them said. "The way the Tourette's disappears." And Bennett himself was astonished, too, and quizzed me, as he peeled off his gloves, on the neurophysiology of it all.

Things were not always so easy, Bennett told me later. Occasionally, if he was bombarded by outside demands during surgery—"You have three patients waiting in the E.R.," "Mrs. X. wants to know if she can come in on the tenth," "Your wife wants you to pick up three bags of dog food"—these pressures, these distractions, would break his concentration, break the smooth and rhythmic flow. A couple of years ago, he made it a rule that he must never be disturbed while operating and must be allowed to concentrate totally on the surgery, and the O.R. has been tic-free ever since.

Bennett's operating brings up all the conundrums of Tourette's, along with deep issues such as the nature of rhythm, melody, and "flow," and the nature of acting, role, personation, and identity. A transition from uncoordinated, jerky ticciness to smooth orchestrated, coherent movement can occur instantly in Touretters when they are exposed to, called into, rhythmic music or action. I saw this with the man I described in "Witty Ticcy Ray," who could swim the length of a pool without tics, with even, rhythmic strokes—but in the instant of turning, when the rhythm, the kinetic melody, was broken, would have a sudden flurry of tics. Many Touretters are also drawn to athletics, partly (one suspects) because of their extraordinary speed and accuracy,[9] and partly because of their bursting, inordinate motor impulse and energy, which thrust toward some motor release—but a release that, happily, instead of being explosive, can be coordinated into the flow, the rhythm, of a performance or a game.

One sees very similar situations with playing or responding to music. The convulsive or broken motor or speech patterns that may occur in Tourette's can be instantly normalized with incanting or singing (this has also long been known

[9] What most of us call a startling or "abnormal" speed of movement appears perfectly normal to Touretters when they show it. This was very clear in a recent experiment of target pointing with Shane F., an artist with Tourette's. Shane showed markedly reduced reaction times, and reaching rates of almost six times normal, combined with great smoothness and accuracy of movement and aim. Such speeds were achieved quite effortlessly and naturally; normal subjects, by contrast, could achieve them, if at all, only by violent effort and with obvious compromise of accuracy and control.

On the other hand, when Shane was asked to stick to (our) normal speeds, his movements became constrained, awkward, inaccurate, and tic filled. It was clear that *his* normal and *our* normal were very different, that the Tourettic nervous system, in this sense, is more highly tuned (though, by the same token, given to precipitancy and reaction).

A similar speed and precipitancy were to be seen in many post-encephalitic patients, especially when they were activated by L-DOPA. Thus, as I remarked of Hester Y., in *Awakenings*, "If Mrs. Y., before L-DOPA was the most *impeded* person I have ever seen, she became, on L-DOPA, the most *accelerated* person I have ever seen. I have known a number of Olympic athletes, but Mrs. Y. could have beaten them all in terms of reaction time; under other circumstances she could have been the fastest gun in the West."

to occur with stutterers). It is similar with the jerky, broken movements of parkinsonism (sometimes called kinetic stutter); these too can be replaced, with music or action, by a rhythmic, melodic flow.

Such responses seem to involve chiefly the motor patterns of the individual, rather than the persona, the identity, in any higher form. *Some* of the transformation while Bennett was operating, I felt, was occurring at this elementary, "musical" level. At this level, Bennett's operating had become automatic; there were, at every moment, a dozen things to attend to, but these were integrated, orchestrated, into a single seamless stream—and one that, like his driving, had become partly automated with time, so that he could chat with the nurses, make jokes, banter, think, while his hands and eyes and brain performed their skilled tasks faultlessly, almost unconsciously.

But above this level, coexisting with it, was a higher, personal one, which has to do with the identity, the role, of a surgeon. Anatomy (and then surgery) have been Bennett's constant loves, lying at the center of his being, and he is most himself, most deeply himself, when he is immersed in his work. His whole personality and demeanor—sometimes nervous and diffident—change when he puts on his surgical mantle, takes on the quiet assurance, the identity, of one who is a master at his work. It seems part of this overall change that the Tourette's vanishes, too. I have seen exactly this in Tourettic actors as well; I know one man, a character actor, who is violently Touretty offstage, but totally free from Tourettisms, totally in role, when he is acting.

Here one is seeing something at a much higher level than the merely rhythmic, quasi-automatic resonance of the motor patterns; one is seeing (however it is to be defined in psychic or neural terms) a fundamental act of incarnation or personation, whereby the skills, the feelings, the entire neural engrams of another self, are taking over in the brain, redefining the person, his whole nervous system, as long as the performance lasts.[10] Such identity transformations, reorganizations, occur in us all as we move, in the course of a day, from one role, one persona, to another— the parental to the professional, to the political, to the erotic, or whatever. But they are especially dramatic in those who move in and out of neurological or psychiatric syndromes, and in professional performers and actors.

These transformations, the switches between very complex neural engrams, are typically experienced in terms of "remembering" and "forgetting"—thus Bennett forgets that he is Tourettic while operating ("it never even crosses my mind"), but remembers it as soon as there is an interruption. And in the moment of remembering, he becomes so, for at this level, there is no distinction between the

[10]The matter is especially complex, for some Touretters are given to mimicry, imitation, and impersonation of a more convulsive kind. (I describe an example of this in "The Possessed.") This sort of imitation has no transformative effect; on the contrary, it thrusts the person deeper into Tourette's. The Tourettic character actor was very given to convulsive impersonations and other Tourettisms offstage, but these were quite different from the deep and healing role-playing that he was able to do onstage. The superficially imitative or impersonative impulse comes from, and stimulates, a superficial part of the person (and his neural organization)—it is only a deep, total identification, as with Bennett, that can work the transformation.

memory, the knowledge, the impulse, and the act—all come
or go together, as one. (It is similar with other conditions: I
once saw a parkinsonian man I know take a shot of apo-
morphine to help his rigidity and "freezing"—he suddenly
unfroze a couple of minutes later, smiled, and said, "I have
forgotten how to be parkinsonian.")

Friday afternoon is open. Bennett often likes to go for long
hikes on Fridays, or cycle rides, or drives, with a sense of
the trail, the open road, before him. There is a favorite
ranch he loves to go to, with a beautiful lake and an
airstrip, accessible only via a rugged dirt road. It is a won-
derfully situated ranch, a narrow fertile strip perfectly
placed between the lake and mountains, and we walked for
miles, talking of this and that, with Bennett botanizing or
geologizing as we went. Then, briefly, we went to the lake,
where I took a swim; when I came out of the water I
found that Bennett, rather suddenly, had curled up for a
nap. He looked peaceful, tension-free, as he slept; and the
suddenness and depth of his sleep made me wonder how
much difficulty he encountered in the daytime, whether
he might not sometimes be stressed to the limit. I wondered
how much he concealed beneath his genial surface—how
much, inwardly, he had to control and deal with.

Later, as we continued our ramble about the ranch, he
remarked that I had seen only some of the outward expres-
sions of his Tourette's, and these, bizarre as they occasionally seemed, were by no means the worst problems it

caused him. The real problems, the inner problems, are panic and rage—feelings so violent that they threaten to overwhelm him, and so sudden that he has virtually no warning of their onset. He has only to get a parking ticket or see a police car, sometimes, for scenarios of violence to flash through his mind: mad chases, shoot-outs, flaming destructions, violent mutilation, and death scenarios that become immensely elaborated in seconds and rush through his mind with convulsive speed. One part of him, uninvolved, can watch these scenes with detachment, but another part of him is taken over and impelled to action. He can prevent himself from giving way to outbursts in public, but the strain of controlling himself is severe and exhausting. At home, in private, he can let himself go— not at others but at inanimate objects around him. There was the wall I had seen, which he had often struck in his rage, and the refrigerator, at which he had flung virtually everything in the kitchen. In his office, he had kicked a hole in the wall and had had to put a plant in front to cover it; and in his study at home the cedar walls were covered with knife marks. "It's not gentle," he said to me. "You can see it as whimsical, funny—be tempted to romanticize it— but Tourette's comes from deep down in the nervous system and the unconscious. It taps into the oldest, strongest feelings we have. Tourette's is like an epilepsy in the subcortex; when it takes over, there's just a thin line of control, a thin line of cortex, between you and it, between you and that raging storm, the blind force of the subcortex. One can see the charming things, the funny things, the creative side of Tourette's, but there's also that dark side. You have to fight it all your life."

Driving back from the ranch was a stimulating, at times terrifying, experience. Now that Bennett was getting to know me, he felt at liberty to let himself and his Tourette's go. The steering wheel was abandoned for seconds at a time— or so it seemed to me, in my alarm—while he tapped on the windshield (to a litany of "Hooty-hoo!" and "Hi, there!" and "Hideous!"), rearranged his glasses, "centered" them in a hundred different ways, and, with bent forefingers, continually smoothed and evened his mustache while gazing in the rearview mirror rather than at the road. His need to center the steering wheel in relation to his knees also grew almost frenetic: he had constantly to "balance" it, to jerk it to and fro, causing the car to zigzag erratically down the road. "Don't worry," he said when he saw my anxiety. "I know this road. I could see from way back that nothing was coming. I've never had an accident driving."[11]

The impulse to look, and to be looked at, is very striking with Bennett, and, indeed, as soon as we got back to the

---

[11]Driving cross-country with another friend with Tourette's was also a memorable experience, for he would twitch the steering wheel violently from side to side, stamp on the brake or the accelerator suddenly, or pull out the ignition key at speed. But he always checked that these Tourettisms were safe, and never had an accident in ten years of driving.

house he seized Mark and planted himself in front of him, smoothing his mustache furiously and saying, "Look at me! Look at me!" Mark, arrested, stayed where he was, but his eyes wandered to and fro. Now Bennett seized Mark's head, held it rigidly toward him, hissing. "Look, look at me!" And Mark became totally still, transfixed, as if hypnotized.

I found this scene disquieting. Other scenes with the family I had found rather moving: Bennett dabbing at Helen's hair, symmetrically, with outstretched fingers, going "whoo, whoo" softly. She was placid, accepting; it was a touching scene, both tender and absurd. "I love him as he is," Helen said. "I wouldn't want him any other way." Bennett feels the same way: "Funny disease—I don't think of it as a disease but as just me. I say the word 'disease,' but it doesn't seem to be the appropriate word."

It is difficult for Bennett, and is often difficult for Touretters, to see their Tourette's as something external to themselves, because many of its tics and urges may be felt as intentional, as an integral part of the self, the personality, the will. It is quite different, by contrast, with something like parkinsonism or chorea: these have no quality of self-ness or intentionality and are always felt as diseases, as outside the self. Compulsions and tics occupy an intermediate position, seeming sometimes to be an expression of one's personal will, sometimes a coercion of it by another, alien will. These ambiguities are often expressed in the terms people use. Thus the separateness of "it" and "I" is sometimes expressed by jocular personifications of the Tourette's: one Touretter I know calls his Tourette's "Toby," another

"Mr. T." By contrast, a Tourettic possession of the self was vividly expressed by one young man in Utah, who wrote to me that he had a "Tourettized soul."

Though Bennett is quite prepared, even eager, to think of Tourette's in neurochemical or neurophysiological terms—he thinks in terms of chemical abnormalities, of "circuits turning on and off," and of "primitive, normally inhibited behaviors being released"—he also feels it as something that has come to be part of himself. For this reason (among others), he has found that he cannot tolerate haloperidol and similar drugs—they reduce his Tourette's, assuredly but they reduce *him* as well, so that he no longer feels fully himself. "The side effects of haloperidol were dreadful," he said. "I was intensely restless, I couldn't stand still, my body twisted, I shuffled like a parkinsonian. It was a huge relief to get off it. On the other hand, Prozac has been a godsend for the obsessions, the rages, though it doesn't touch the tics." Prozac has indeed been a godsend for many Touretters, though some have found it to have no effect, and a few have had paradoxical effects—an intensification of their agitations, obsessions, and rages.[12]

Though Bennett has had tics since the age of seven or so, he did not identify what he had as Tourette's syndrome until he was thirty-seven. "When we were first married, he just called it a 'nervous habit,'" Helen told me. "We used

---

[12]This was very clear with another Tourettic physician, an obstetrician, who had not only tics but panics and rages that, with a great effort, he could contain. When he was put on Prozac, this precarious control broke down, and he got into a violent fight with the police and spent a night in jail.

to joke about it. I'd say, 'I'll quit smoking, and you quit twitching.' We thought of it as something he *could* quit if he wanted. You'd ask him, 'Why do you do it?' He'd say, 'I don't know why.' He didn't seem to be self-conscious about it. Then, in 1977, when Mark was a baby, Carl heard this program, 'Quirks and Quarks,' on the radio. He got all excited and hollered, 'Helen, come listen! This guy's talking about what I do!' He was excited to hear that other people had it. And it was a relief to me, because I had always sensed that there was something wrong. It was good to put a label on it. He never made a thing of it, he wouldn't raise the subject, but, once we knew, we'd tell people if they asked. It's only in the last few years that he's met other people with it, or gone to meetings of the Tourette Syndrome Association." (Tourette's syndrome, until very recently, was remarkably underdiagnosed and unknown, even to the medical profession, and most people diagnosed themselves, or were diagnosed by friends and family, after seeing or reading something about it in the media. Indeed, I know of another doctor, a surgeon in Louisiana, who was diagnosed by one of his own patients who had seen a Touretter on the Phil Donahue show. Even now, nine out of ten diagnoses are made, not by physicians, but by others who have learned about it from the media. Much of this media emphasis has been due to the efforts of the TSA, which had only thirty members in the early seventies but now has more than twenty thousand.)

Saturday morning, and I have to return to New York. "I'll fly you to Calgary if the weather's fine," Bennett said suddenly last night. "Ever flown with a Touretter before?"

I had canoed with one,[13] I said, and driven across country with another, but flying with one . . .

"You'll enjoy it," Bennett said. "It'll be a novel experience. I am the world's only flying Touretter-surgeon."

When I awake, at dawn, I perceive, with mixed feelings, that the weather, though very cold, is perfect. We drive to the little airport in Branford, a veering, twitching journey that makes me nervous about the flight. "It's much easier in the air, where there's no road to keep to, and you don't have to keep your hands on the controls all the time," Bennett says. At the airport, he parks, opens a hangar, and proudly points out his airplane—a tiny red-and-white single-engine Cessna Cardinal. He pulls it out onto the tarmac and then checks it, rechecks it, and re-rechecks it before warming up the engine. It is near freezing on the airfield, and a north wind is blowing. I watch all the checks and rechecks with impatience but also with a sense of reassurance. If his Tourette's makes him check everything three or five times, so much the safer. I had a similar feeling of reassurance about his surgery—that his Tourette's, if anything,

---

[13] Canoeing with Shane F. one summer on Lake Huron was a remarkable human and clinical experience, for the canoe became an extension of his body, would pitch and plunge with each of his Tourettisms, giving me an unforgettably direct sense of what it must be like to be him. We were constantly flung around, as in a storm, constantly on the point of overturning, and I longed for the canoe to founder, and sink once and for all, so that I could escape and swim back to the shore.

made him more meticulous, more exact, without in the least damping down his intuitiveness, his freedom.

His checking done, Bennett leaps like a trapeze artist into the plane, revs the engine while I climb in, and takes off. As we climb, the sun is rising over the Rockies to the east and floods the little cabin with a pale, golden light. We head toward nine-thousand-foot crests, and Bennett tics, flutters, reaches, taps, touches his glasses, his mustache, the top of the cockpit. Minor tics, Little League, I think, but what if he has big tics? What if he wants to twirl the plane in midair, to hop and skip with it, to do somersaults, to loop the loop? What if he has an impulse to leap out and touch the propeller? Touretters tend to be fascinated by spinning objects; I have a vision of him lunging forward, half out the window, compulsively lunging at the propeller before us. But his tics and compulsions remain very minor, and when he takes his hands off the controls the plane continues quietly. Mercifully, there is no road to keep to. If we rise or fall or veer fifty feet, what does it matter? We have the whole sky to play with.

And Bennett, though superbly skilled, a natural aviator, *is* like a child at play. Part of Tourette's, at least, is no more than this—the release of a playful impulse normally inhibited or lost in the rest of us. The freedom, the spaciousness, obviously delight Bennett; he has a carefree, boyish look I rarely saw on the ground. Now, rising, we fly over the first peaks, the advance guard of the Rockies; yellowing larches stream beneath us. We clear the slopes by a thousand feet or more. I wonder whether Bennett, if he were by himself, might want to clear the peaks by ten feet, by inches—Touretters are sometimes addicted to close shaves. At ten thousand feet, we move in a corridor between peaks, mountains shining in the morning sun to our left, mountains silhouetted against it to our right. At eleven thousand feet, we can see the whole width of the Rockies—they are only fifty-five miles across here—and the vast golden Alberta prairie starting to the east. Every so often Bennett's right arm flashes in front of me, his hand taps lightly on the windshield. "Sedimentary rocks, look!" He gestures through the window. "Lifted up from the sea bottom at seventy to eighty degrees." He gazes at the steeply sloping rocks as at a friend; he is intensely at home with these mountains, this land. Snow lies on the sunless slopes of the mountains, none yet on their sunlit faces; and over to the northwest, toward Banff, we can see glaciers on the mountains. Bennett shifts, and shifts, and shifts again, trying to get his knees exactly symmetrical beneath the controls of the plane.

In Alberta now—we have been flying for forty minutes—the Highwood River winds beneath us. Flying due north, we start a gentle descent toward Calgary, the last, declining slopes of the Rockies all shimmering with aspen. Now, lower, to vast fields of wheat and alfalfa—farms, ranches, fertile prairie—but still, everywhere, stands of golden aspen. Beyond the checkerboard of fields, the towers of Calgary rise abruptly from the flat plain.

Suddenly, the radio crackles alive—a huge Russian air transport is coming in; the main runway, closed for maintenance, must quickly be opened up. Another massive plane, from the Zambian air force. The world's planes come to Calgary for special work and maintenance; its facilities, Bennett tells me, are some of the best in North America. In the middle of this important flurry, Bennett radios in our position and statistics (fifteen-feet-long Cardinal, with a Touretter and his neurologist) and is immediately answered, as fully and helpfully as if he were a 747. All planes, all pilots, are equal in this world. And it is a world apart, with a freemasonry of its own, its own language, codes, myths, and manners. Bennett, clearly, is part of this world and is recognized by the traffic controller and greeted cheerfully as he taxis in.

He leaps out with a startling, ticlike suddenness and celerity—I follow at a slower, "normal" pace—and starts talking with two giant young men on the tarmac, Kevin and Chuck, brothers, both fourth-generation pilots in the Rockies. They know him well. "He's just one of us," Chuck says to me. "A regular guy. Tourette's—what the hell? He's a good human being. A damn good pilot, too."

Bennett yarns with his fellow pilots and files his flight plan for the return trip to Branford. He has to return straightaway; he is due to speak at eleven to a group of nurses, and his subject, for once, is not surgery but Tourette's. His little plane is refueled and readied for the return flight. We hug and say good-bye, and as I head for my flight to New York I turn to watch him go. Bennett walks to his plane, taxis onto the main runway, and takes off, fast, with a tailwind following. I watch him for a while, and then he is gone.

# THE VISIONS OF HILDEGARD

The religious literature of all ages is replete with descriptions of "visions," in which sublime and ineffable feelings have been accompanied by the experience of radiant luminosity (William James speaks of "photism" in this context). It is impossible to ascertain, in the vast majority of cases, whether the experience represents a hysterical or psychotic ecstasy, the effects of intoxication, or an epileptic or migrainous manifestation. A unique exception is provided in the case of Hildegard of Bingen (1098 to 1180), a nun and mystic of exceptional intellectual and literary powers, who experienced countless "visions" from earliest childhood to the close of her life, and has left exquisite accounts and figures of these in the two manuscript codices which have come down to us—*Scivias* and *Liber divinorum operum simplicis hominis.*

A careful consideration of these accounts and figures

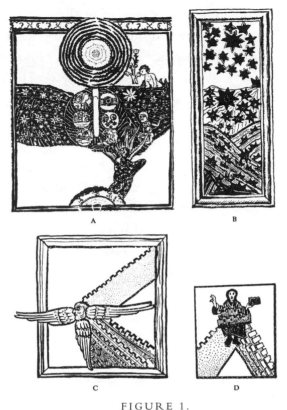

FIGURE 1.

*Varieties of migraine hallucination represented in the visions of Hildegard*

Representations of migrainous visions, from a MS. of Hildegard's *Scivias*, written at Bingen about 1180. In Figure 1A, the background is formed of shimmering stars set upon wavering concentric lines. In Figure 1B a shower of brilliant stars (phosphenes) is extinguished after its passage—the succession of positive and negative scotoma: in Figures 1C and 1D, Hildegard depicts typically migrainous fortification figures radiating from a central point, which, in the original, is brilliantly luminous and coloured (see text).

leaves no room for doubt concerning their nature: they were indisputably migrainous, and they illustrate, indeed, many of the varieties of visual aura earlier discussed. Singer (1958), in the course of an extensive essay on Hildegard's visions, selects the following phenomena as most characteristic of them:

> In all a prominent feature is a point or a group of points of light, which shimmer and move, usually in a wave-like manner, and are most often interpreted as stars of flaming eyes. In quite a number of cases one light, larger than the rest, exhibits a series of concentric circular figures of wavering form; and often definite fortification figures are described, radiating in some cases from a coloured area. Often the lights gave that impression of *working*, boiling or fermenting, described by so many visionaries . . .

Hildegard writes:

> The visions which I saw I beheld neither in sleep, not in dreams, nor in madness, nor with my carnal eyes, nor with the ears of the flesh, nor in hidden places; but wakeful alert, and with the eyes of the spirit and the inward ears, I perceived them in open view and according to the will of God.

One such vision, illustrated by a figure of stars falling and being quenched in the ocean signifies for her "The Fall of the Angels":

I saw a great star most splendid and beautiful, and with it an exceeding multitude of falling stars which with the star followed southwards . . . And suddenly they were all annihilated, being turned into black coals . . . and cast into the abyss so that I could see them no more.

Such is Hildegard's allegorical interpretation. Our literal interpretation would be that she experienced a shower of phosphenes in transit across the visual field, their passage being succeeded by a negative scotoma. Visions with fortification-figures are represented in her *Zelus Dei* (Figure 1C) and *Sedens Lucidus* (Figure 1D), the fortifications radiating from a brilliantly luminous and (in the original) shimmering and coloured point. These two visions are combined in a composite vision, and in this she interprets the fortifications as the *aedificium* of the city of God.

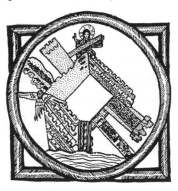

"Vision of the Heavenly City"

Great rapturous intensity invests the experience of these auras, especially on the rare occasions when a second scotoma follows in the wake of the original scintillation:

The light which I see is not located, but yet is more brilliant than the sun, nor can I examine its height, length or breadth, and I name it "the cloud of the living light." And as sun, moon, and stars are reflected in water, so the writings, sayings, virtues and works of men shine in it before me. . . .

Sometimes I behold within this light another light which I name "the Living Light itself." . . . And when I look upon it every sadness and pain vanishes from my memory, so that I am again as a simple maid and not as an old woman.

Invested with this sense of ecstasy, burning with profound theophorous and philosophical significance, Hildegard's visions were instrumental in directing her toward a life of holiness and mysticism. They provide a unique example of the manner in which a physiological event, banal, hateful, or meaningless to the vast majority of people, can become, in a privileged consciousness, the substrate of a supreme ecstatic inspiration. One must go to Dostoevski, who experienced on occasion ecstatic epileptic auras to which he attached momentous significance, to find an adequate historical parallel.[1]

[1] "There are moments [Dostoevski writes of such auras], and it is only a matter of five or six seconds, when you feel the presence of the eternal harmony . . . a terrible thing is the frightful clearness with which it manifests itself and the rapture with which it fills you. If this state were to last more than five seconds, the soul could not endure it and would have to disappear. During these five seconds I live a whole human existence, and for that I would give my whole life and not think that I was paying too dearly. . . ."

# ISLAND HOPPING

As a child I had visual migraines, where I would have not only the classical scintillations and alterations of the visual field, but alterations in the sense of color too, which might weaken or entirely disappear for a few minutes. This experience frightened me, but tantalized me too, and made me wonder what it would be like to live in a completely colorless world, not just for a few minutes, but permanently. It was not until many years later that I got an answer, at least a partial answer, in the form of a patient, Jonathan I., a painter who had suddenly become totally colorblind following a car accident (and perhaps a stroke). He had lost color vision not through any damage to his eyes, it seemed, but through damage to the parts of the brain which "construct" the sensation of color. Indeed, he

The text of this selection has been edited slightly from its original form in *The Island of the Colorblind*.

seemed to have lost the ability not only to see color, but to imagine or remember it, even to dream of it. Nevertheless, like an amnesic, he in some way remained conscious of having *lost* color, after a lifetime of chromatic vision, and complained of his world feeling impoverished, grotesque, abnormal—his art, his food, even his wife looked "leaden" to him. Still, he could not assuage my curiosity on the allied, yet totally different, matter of what it might be like *never* to have seen color, never to have had the least sense of its primal quality, its place in the world.

Ordinary colorblindness, arising from a defect in the retinal cells, is almost always partial, and some forms are very common: red-green colorblindness occurs to some degree in one in twenty men (it is much rarer in women). But total congenital colorblindness, or achromatopsia, is surpassingly rare, affecting perhaps only one person in thirty or forty thousand. What, I wondered, would the visual world be like for those born totally colorblind? Would they, perhaps, lacking any sense of something missing, have a world no less dense and vibrant than our own? Might they even have developed heightened perceptions of visual tone and texture and movement and depth, and live in a world in some ways more intense than our own, a world of heightened reality—one that we can only glimpse echoes of in the work of the great black-and-white photographers? Might they indeed see *us* as peculiar, distracted by trivial or irrelevant aspects of the visual world, and insufficiently sensitive to its real visual essence? I could only guess, as I had never met anyone born completely colorblind.

Knowing that congenital achromatopsia is hereditary, I could not help wondering whether there might be, somewhere on the planet, an island, a village, a valley of the colorblind. When I visited Guam early in 1993, some impulse made me put this question to my friend John Steele, who has practiced neurology all over Micronesia. Unexpectedly, I received an immediate, positive answer: there *was* just such an isolate, John said, on the island of Pingelap—it was relatively close, "barely twelve hundred miles from here," he added. Just a few days earlier, he had seen an achromatopic boy on Guam, who had journeyed there with his parents from Pingelap. "Fascinating," he said. "Classical congenital achromatopsia, with nystagmus, and avoidance of bright light—and the incidence on Pingelap is extraordinarily high, almost ten percent of the population." I was intrigued by what John told me, and resolved that—sometime—I would come back to the South Seas and visit Pingelap.

When I returned to New York, the thought receded to the back of my mind. Then, some months later, I got a long letter from Frances Futterman, a woman in Berkeley who was herself born completely colorblind. She had read my essay on the colorblind painter and was at pains to contrast her situation with his, and to emphasize that she herself, never having known color, had no sense of loss, no sense of being chromatically defective. But congenital achromatopsia, she pointed out, involved far more than colorblindness as such. What was far more disabling was the painful hypersensitivity to light and poor visual acuity which also affect congenital achromatopes. She had grown up in a relatively shadeless part of Texas, with a constant squint, and preferred to go out only at night. She was intrigued by the notion of an island of the colorblind, and wondered if I knew of a book called *Night Vision*—one of its editors, she added, was an achromatope too, a Norwegian scientist name Knut Nordby; perhaps he could tell me more.

Knut Nordby was a physiologist and psychophysicist, I read, a vision researcher at the University of Oslo and, partly by virtue of his own condition, an expert on colorblindness. This was surely a unique, and important, combination of personal and formal knowledge; I had also sensed a warm, open quality in his brief autobiographical memoir, which forms a chapter of *Night Vision*, and this emboldened me to write to him in Norway, asking how he might feel about coming with me on a ten-thousand-mile journey, a sort of scientific adventure to Pingelap, and he replied yes, he would love to come, and could take off a few weeks in August.

I asked my friend and colleague Robert Wasserman if he would join us as well. As an ophthalmologist, Bob sees many partially colorblind people in his practice. Like myself, he had never met anyone born totally colorblind;

but we had worked together on several cases involving vision, including that of the colorblind painter, Mr. I. As young doctors, we had done fellowships in neuropathology together, back in the 1960s, and I remembered him telling me then of his four-year-old son, Eric, as they drove up to Maine one summer, exclaiming, "Look at the beautiful orange grass!" No, Bob told him, it's not orange— "orange" is the color of an orange. Yes, cried Eric, it's orange like an orange! This was Bob's first intimation of his son's colorblindness. Later, when he was six, Eric had painted a picture he called *The Battle of Grey Rock*, but had used pink pigment for the rock.

Bob, as I had hoped, was fascinated by the prospect of meeting Knut and voyaging to Pingelap. An ardent windsurfer and sailor, he has a passion for oceans and islands and is reconditely knowledgeable about the evolution of outrigger canoes and proas in the Pacific; he longed to see these in action, to sail one himself. Along with Knut, we would form a team, an expedition at once neurological, scientific, and romantic, to the Caroline archipelago and the island of the colorblind.

# PINGELAP

Pingelap is one of eight tiny atolls scattered in the ocean around Pohnpei. Once lofty volcanic islands like Pohnpei, they are geologically much older and have eroded and subsided over millions of years, leaving only rings of coral surrounding lagoons, so that the combined area of all the atolls—Ant, Pakin, Nukuoro, Oroluk, Kapingamarangi, Mwoakil, Sapwuahfik, and Pingelap—is now no more than three square miles. Though Pingelap is one of the farthest from Pohnpei, 180 miles (of often rough seas) distant, it was settled before the other atolls, a thousand years ago, and still has the largest population, about seven hundred. There is not much commerce or communication between the islands, and only a single boat plying the route between them: the MS *Microglory*, which ferries cargo and occa-

The text of this selection has been edited slightly from its original form in *The Island of the Colorblind.*

sional passengers, making its circuit (if wind and sea permit) five or six times a year.

Since the *Microglory* was not due to leave for another month, we chartered a tiny prop plane run by the Pacific Missionary Aviation service; it was flown by a retired commercial airliner pilot from Texas who now lived in Pohnpei. We barely managed to squeeze ourselves in, along with luggage, ophthalmoscope and various testing materials, snorkeling gear, photographic and recording equipment, and special extra supplies for the achromatopes: two hundred pairs of sunglass visors, of varying darkness and hue, plus a smaller number of infant sunglasses and shades.

The plane, specially designed for the short island runways, was slow, but had a reassuring, steady drone, and we flew low enough to see shoals of tuna in the water. It was an hour before we sighted the atoll of Mwoakil, and another hour before we saw the three islets of Pingelap atoll, forming a broken crescent around the lagoon.

We flew twice around the atoll to get a closer view—a view which at first disclosed nothing but unbroken forest. It was only when we skimmed the trees, two hundred feet from the ground, that we could make out paths intersecting the forest here and there, and low houses almost hidden in the foliage.

Very suddenly, the wind rose—it had been tranquil a few minutes before—and the coconut palms and pandanus trees began lashing to and fro. As we made for the tiny concrete airstrip at one end, built by the occupying Japanese a half century before, a violent tailwind seized us near the ground, and almost blew us off the side of the runway. Our pilot struggled to control the skidding plane, for now, having just missed the edge of the landing strip, we were in danger of shooting off the end. By main force, and luck, he just managed to bring the plane around—another six inches and we would have been in the lagoon. "You folks OK?" he asked us, and then, to himself, "Worst landing I ever had!"

Knut and Bob were ashen, the pilot too—they had visions of being submerged in the plane, struggling, suffocating, unable to get out; I myself felt a curious indifference, even a sense that it would be fun, romantic, to die on the reef— and then a sudden, huge wave of nausea. But even in our extremity, as the brakes screamed to halt us, I seemed to hear laughter, sounds of mirth, all around us. As we got out, still pale with shock, dozens of lithe brown children ran out of the forest, waving flowers, banana leaves, laughing, surrounding us. I could see no adults at first, and thought for a moment that Pingelap was an island of children. And in that first long moment, with the children coming out of the forest, some with their arms around each other, and the tropical luxuriance of vegetation in all directions—the beauty of the primitive, the human and the natural, took hold of me. I felt a wave of love—for the children, for the forest, for the island, for the whole scene; I had a sense of paradise, of an almost magical reality. I thought, I have arrived. I am here at last. I want to spend the rest of my life here—and some of these beautiful children could be mine.

"Beautiful!" whispered Knut, enraptured, by my side,

and then, "Look at that child—and that one, and that. . . ."
I followed his glance, and now suddenly saw what I had
first missed: here and there, among the rest, clusters of
children who squinted, screwed up their eyes against the
bright sun, and one, an older boy, with a black cloth over
his head. Knut had seen them, identified them, his achromatopic brethren, the moment he stepped out of the
plane—as they, clearly, spotted him the moment he stepped
out, squinting, dark-glassed, by the side of the plane.

Though Knut had read the scientific literature, and
though he had occasionally met other achromatopic people,
this had in no way prepared him for the impact of actually
finding himself surrounded by his own kind, strangers half
a world away with whom he had an instant kinship. It was
an odd sort of encounter which the rest of us were wit-
nessing—pale, Nordic Knut in his Western clothes, camera
around his neck, and the small brown achromatopic children of Pingelap—but intensely moving.[1]

Eager hands grabbed our luggage, while our equipment
was loaded onto an improvised trolley—an unstable con-

---

[1] A similar feeling of kinship may occur for a deaf traveler, who has crossed the
sea or the world, if he lights upon other deaf people on his arrival. In 1814, the
deaf French educator Laurent Clerc came to visit a deaf school in London, and
this was described by a contemporary:

> As soon as Clerc beheld this sight [of the children at dinner] his face
> became animated: he was as agitated as a traveller of sensibility would
> be on meeting all of a sudden in distant regions, a colony of his coun-
> trymen. . . . Clerc approached them. He made signs and they answered
> him by signs. This unexpected communication caused a most delicious
> sensation in them and for us was a scene of expression and sensibility
> that gave us the most heartfelt satisfaction.                    (*cont.*)

traption of rough-hewn planks on trembling bicycle wheels. There are no powered vehicles on Pingelap, no paved roads, only trodden-earth or graveled paths through the woods, all connecting, directly or indirectly, with the main drag, a broader tract with houses to either side, some tin-roofed, and some thatched with leaves. It was on this main path that we were now being taken, escorted by dozens of excited children and young adults (we had seen no one, as yet, over twenty-five or thirty).

Our arrival—with sleeping bags, bottled water, medical and film equipment—was an event almost without precedent (the island children were fascinated not so much by our cameras as by the sound boom with its woolly muff, and within a day were making their own booms out of banana stalks and coconut wool). There was a lovely festive quality to this spontaneous procession, which had no order, no program, no leader, no precedence, just a raggle-taggle of wondering, gaping people (they at us, we at them and everything around us), making our way, with many

---

And it was similar when I went with Lowell Handler, a friend with Tourette's syndrome, to a remote Mennonite community in northern Alberta where a genetic form of Tourette's had become remarkably common. At first a bit tense, and on his best behavior, Lowell was able to suppress his tics; but after a few minutes he let out a loud Tourettic shriek. Everyone turned to look at him, as always happens. But then everybody smiled—they understood—and some even answered Lowell with their own tics and noises. Surrounded by other Touretters, his Tourettic brethren, Lowell felt, in many ways, that he had "come home" at last—he dubbed the village "Tourettesville," and mused about marrying a beautiful Mennonite woman with Tourette's, and living there happily ever after.

stops and diversions and detours, through the forest-village of Pingelap. Little black-and-white piglets darted across our path—unshy, but unaffectionate, unpetlike too, leading their own seemingly autonomous existence, as if the island were equally theirs. We were struck by the fact that the pigs were black and white and wondered, half seriously, if they had been specially bred for, or by, an achromatopic population.

None of us voiced this thought aloud, but our interpreter, James James, himself achromatopic—a gifted young man, who (unlike most of the islanders) had spent a considerable time off-island and been educated at the University of Guam—read our glances and said, "Our ancestors brought these pigs when they came to Pingelap a thousand years ago, as they brought the breadfruit and yams, and the myths and rituals of our people."

Although the pigs scampered wherever there was food (they were evidently fond of bananas and rotted mangoes and coconuts), they were all, James told us, individually owned—and, indeed, could be counted as an index of the owner's material status and prosperity. Pigs were originally a royal food, and no one but the king, the nahnmwarki, might eat them; even now they were slaughtered rarely, mostly on special ceremonial occasions.

Knut was fascinated not only by the pigs but by the richness of the vegetation, which he saw quite clearly, perhaps more clearly than the rest of us. For us, as color-normals, it was at first just a confusion of greens, whereas to Knut it was a polyphony of brightnesses, tonalities, shapes, and textures, easily identified and distinguished from each other. He mentioned this to James, who said it was the same for him, for all the achromatopes on the island— none of them had any difficulty distinguishing the plants on the island. He thought they were helped in this, perhaps, by the basically monchrome nature of the landscape: there were a few red flowers and fruits on the island, and these, it was true, they might miss in certain lighting situations—but virtually all else was green.[2]

---

[2]It was striking how green everything was in Pingelap, not only the foliage of trees, but their fruits as well—breadfruit and pandanus are both green, as were many varieties of bananas on the island. The brightly colored red and yellow fruits—papaya, mango, guava—are not native to these islands, but were only introduced by the Europeans in the 1820s.

J. D. Mollon, a preeminent researcher on the mechanisms of color vision, notes that Old World monkeys "are particularly attracted to orange or yellow fruit (as opposed to birds, which go predominantly for red or purple fruit)." Most mammals (indeed, most vertebrates) have evolved a system of dichromatic vision, based on the correlation of short- and medium-wavelength information, which helps them to recognize their environments, their foods, their friends and enemies, and to live in a world of color, albeit of a very limited and muted type. Only certain primates have evolved full trichromatic vision, and this is what enables them to detect yellow and orange fruits against a dappled green background; Mollon suggests that the coloration of these fruits may indeed have coevolved with such a trichromatic system in monkeys. Trichromatic vision enables them too to recognize the most delicate facial shades of emotional and biological states, and to use these (as monkeys do, no less than humans) to signal aggression or sexual display.

Achromatopes, or rod-monochromats (as they are also called), lack even the primordial dichromatic system, considered to have developed far back in the Paleozoic. If "human dichromats," in Mollon's words, "have especial difficulty in detecting colored fruit against dappled foliage that varies randomly in luminosity," one would expect that monochromats would be even more profoundly disabled, scarcely able to survive in a world geared, at the least, for

"But what about bananas, let's say—can you distinguish the yellow from the green ones?" Bob asked.

"Not always," James replied. " 'Pale green' may look the same to me as 'yellow.' "

"How can you tell when a banana is ripe, then?"

James' answer was to go to banana tree, and to come back with a carefully selected, bright green banana for Bob.

Bob peeled it; it peeled easily, to his surprise. He took a small bite of it, gingerly; then devoured the rest.

"You see," said James, "we don't just go by color. We look, we feel, we smell, we *know*—we take everything into consideration, and you just take color!"

I had seen the general shape of Pingelap from the air— three islets forming a broken ring around a central lagoon

---

dichromats. But it is here that adaptation and compensation can play a crucial part. This quite different mode of perception is well brought out by Frances Futterman, who writes:

> When a new object would come into my life, I would have a very thorough sensory experience of it. I would savor the feel of it, the smell of it, and the appearance of it (all the visible aspects except color, of course). I would even stroke it or tap it or do whatever created an auditory experience. All objects have unique qualities which can be savored. All can be looked at in different lights and in different kinds of shadows. Dull finishes, shiny finishes, textures, prints, transparent qualities—I scrutinized them all, up close, in my accustomed way (which occurred because of my visual impairment but which, I think, provided me with more multi-sensory impressions of things). How might this have been different if I were seeing in color? Might the colors of things have dominated my experience, preventing me from knowing so intimately the other qualities of things?

perhaps a mile and a half in diameter; now, walking on a narrow strip of land, with the crashing surf to one side and the tranquil lagoon only a few hundred yards to the other, I was reminded of the absolute awe that seized the early explorers who had first come upon these alien land forms, so utterly unlike anything in their experience. "It is a marvel," wrote Pyrard de Laval in 1605, "to see each of these atolls, surrounded by a great bank of stone involving no human artifice at all."

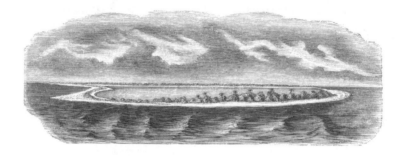

Cook, sailing the Pacific, was intrigued by these low atolls, and could already, in 1777, speak of the puzzlement and controversy surrounding them:

Some will have it they are the remains of large islands, that in remote times were joined and formed one continued track of land which the Sea in process of time has washed away and left only the higher grounds. . . . Others and I think . . . that they are formed from Shoals or Coral banks and of consequence increasing; and there are some who think they have been thrown up by Earth quakes.

But by the beginning of the nineteenth century it had become clear that while coral atolls might emerge in the deepest parts of the ocean, the living coral itself could not grow more than a hundred feet or so below the surface and had to have a firm foundation at this depth. Thus it was not imaginable, as Cook conceived, that sediments or corals could build up from the ocean floor.

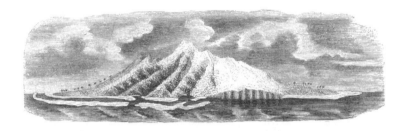

Sir Charles Lyell, the supreme geologist of his age, postulated that atolls were the coral-encrusted rims of rising submarine volcanoes, but this seemed to require an almost impossible serendipity of innumerable volcanoes thrusting up to within fifty or eighty feet of the surface to provide a platform for the coral, without ever actually breaking the surface.

Darwin, on the Chilean coast, had experienced at first hand the huge cataclysms of earthquakes and volcanoes; these, for him, were "parts of one of the greatest phenom-

ena to which this world is subject"—notably, the instabil-
ity, the continuous movements, the geological oscillations
of the earth's crust. Images of vast risings and sinkings
seized his imagination: the Andes rising thousands of feet
into the air, the Pacific floor sinking thousands of feet
beneath the surface. And in the context of this general
vision, a specific vision came to him—that such risings and
fallings could explain the origin of oceanic islands, and
their subsidence to allow the formation of coral atolls.
Reversing, in a way, the Lyellian notion, he postulated that
coral grew not on the summits of rising volcanoes, but on
their submerging slopes; then, as the volcanic rock eventually eroded and subsided into the sea, only the coral fringes
remained, forming a barrier reef. As the volcano continued
to subside, new layers of coral polyps could continue to
build upward, now in the characteristic atoll shape, toward
the light and warmth they depended on. The development
of such an atoll would require, he reckoned, at least a million years.

Darwin cited short-term evidence of this subsidence—
palm trees and buildings, for instance, formerly on dry
land, which were now under water; but he realized that
conclusive proof for so slow a geologic process would be
far from easy to obtain. Indeed, his theory (though accepted
by many) was not confirmed until a century later, when an
immense borehole was drilled through the coral of Eniwe-
tak atoll, finally hitting volcanic rock 4,500 feet below the
surface. The reef-constructing corals, for Darwin, were

wonderful memorials of the subterranean oscillations of level . . . each atoll a monument over an island now lost. We may thus, like unto a geologist who had lived his ten thousand years and kept a record of the passing changes, gain some insight into the great system by which the surface of this globe has been broken up, and land and water interchanged.

Looking at Pingelap, thinking of the lofty volcano it once was, sinking infinitesimally slowly for tens of millions of years, I felt an almost tangible sense of the vastness of time, and that our expedition to the South Seas was not only a journey in space, but a journey in time as well.

The sudden wind which had almost blown us off the landing strip was dying down now, although the tops of the palms were still whipping to and fro, and we could still hear the thunder of the surf, pounding the reef in huge rolling breakers. The typhoons which are notorious in this part of the Pacific can be especially devastating to a coral atoll like Pingelap (which is nowhere more than ten feet above sea level)—for the entire island can be inundated, submerged by the huge wind-lashed seas. Typhoon Lengkieki, which swept over Pingelap around 1775, killed 90 percent of the island's population outright, and most of the survivors went on to die a lingering death from starvation—for all the vegetation, even the coconut palms and breadfruit and banana trees, was destroyed, leaving nothing to sustain the islanders but fish.

At the time of the typhoon, Pingelap had a population of nearly a thousand, and had been settled for eight hundred years. It is not known where the original settlers came from, but they brought with them an elaborate hierarchical system ruled by hereditary kings or nahnmwarkis, an oral culture and mythology, and a language which had already differentiated so much by this time that it was hardly intelligible to the "mainlanders" on Pohnpei. This thriving culture was reduced, within a few weeks of the typhoon, to twenty or so survivors, including the nahnmwarki and other members of the royal household.

The Pingelapese are extremely fertile, and within a few decades the population was reapproaching a hundred. But with this heroic breeding—and, of necessity, inbreeding—new problems arose, genetic traits previously rare began to spread, so that in the fourth generation after the typhoon a "new" disease showed itself. The first children with the Pingelap eye disease were born in the 1820s, and within a few generations their numbers had increased to more than five percent of the population, roughly what it remains today.

The mutation for achromatopsia may have arisen among the Carolinians centuries before; but this was a recessive gene, and as long as there was a large enough population the chances of two carriers marrying, and of the condition becoming manifest in their children, were very small. All this altered with the typhoon, and genealogical studies indicate that it was the surviving nahnmwarki himself who was the ultimate progenitor of every subsequent carrier.[3]

Infants with the eye disease appeared normal at birth, but when two or three months old would start to squint or blink, to screw up their eyes or turn their heads away in the face of bright light; and when they were toddlers it became apparent that they could not see fine detail or small objects at a distance. By the time they reached four or five, it was clear they could not distinguish colors. The term maskun ("not-see") was coined to describe this strange condition, which occurred with equal frequency in both male and female children, children otherwise normal, bright, and active in all ways.

Today, over two hundred years after the typhoon, a third of the population are carriers of the gene for maskun, and out of some seven hundred islanders, fifty-seven are achromats. Elsewhere in the world, the incidence of achromatopsia is less than one in thirty thousand—here on Pingelap it is one in twelve.

---

[3]In a small, isolated or recently founded population, accurate geneologies—as preserved orally among the Pingelapese and in written records by many other communities—may make it possible to delineate a single ancestral individual, or a small number of ancestors, as responsible for the spread of a genetic trait; such a situation is referred to by geneticists as "the founder effect." Carefully kept records on Martha's Vineyard show the "founders" of hereditary deafness there to have been two brothers carrying a recessive gene for the trait, who arrived in the 1690s. Similarly, in the little Mennonite community of LaCrete, in Alberta, where there is a high incidence of Tourette's syndrome, all known cases of the disorder can be traced to one Gerhard Jantzen, who arrived from the Ukraine in the 1880s and founded the LaCrete community—with three

Our ragged procession, tipping and swaying through the forest, with children romping and pigs under our feet, finally arrived at the island's administration building, one of the three or four two-story cinderblock buildings on the island. Here we met and were ceremoniously greeted by the nahnmwarki, the magistrate, and other officials. A Pingelapese woman, Delihda Isaac, acted as interpreter, introducing us all, and then herself—she ran the medical dispensary across the way, where she treated all sorts of

---

successive wives, he fathered twenty-four children. And Huntington's chorea in this country can be traced to two (very fertile) brothers arriving on Long Island in the 1630s.

Such genetically (but not necessarily clinically) abnormal individuals would not have so disproportionate an effect in a larger community—but in a small or isolated community, or one proscribing marriage outside the community (as with Mennonites, Amish, Ashkenazi Jews, etc.) there will necessarily be a great deal of intermarriage between blood relatives, many of them (in subsequent generations) now carriers of the gene. A marriage between two such carriers of a recessive gene will be likely to produce some children with manifest disease, in a Mendelian ratio.

Jared Diamond has discussed the founder effect in relation to the changing genetic profile of the world, which has moved, over the last few thousand years, to mixed and genetically homogenized populations—first with the spread of agriculture, then with the establishment of political states, and now with the extreme facility, the incontinence, of world travel. "Human genetic diversity," he writes (in a review of this book):

> must have been much higher in the past than at present, as new populations were constantly being founded and expanding to carry their private genes over small local areas. Pingelap and New Guinea [it was in New Guinea that Diamond's own evolutionary work was first done] are thus far more important to geneticists than their tiny fraction of the world's population would suggest, because they show us our genetic landscape as it used to be.

injuries and illnesses. A few days earlier, she said, she had delivered a breech baby—a difficult job with no medical equipment to speak of—but both mother and child were doing fine. There is no doctor on Pingelap, but Delihda had been educated off-island and was often assisted by trainees from Pohnpei. Any medical problems which she cannot handle have to wait for the visiting nurse from Pohnpei, who makes her rounds to all the outlying islands once a month. But Delihda, Bob observed, though kind and gentle, was clearly a "real force to be reckoned with."

She took us on a brief tour of the administration building—many of the rooms were deserted and empty, and the old kerosene generator designed to light it looked as if it had been out of action for years.[4] As dusk fell, Delihda led the way to the magistrate's house, where we would be quartered. There were no streetlights, no lights anywhere, and the darkness seemed to gather and fall very rapidly. Inside the house, made of concrete blocks, it was dark and small and stiflingly hot, a sweatbox, even after nightfall. But it had a charming outdoor terrace, over which arched a gigantic breadfruit tree and a banana tree. There were two bedrooms—Knut took the magistrate's room below, Bob and I the children's room above. We gazed at each other

---

[4]There are two kerosene generators on Pingelap: one for lighting the administration building and dispensary and three or four other buildings, and one for running the island's videotape recorders. But the first has been out of action for years, and nobody has made much effort to repair or replace it—candles or kerosene lamps are more reliable. The other dynamo, however, is carefully tended, because the viewing of action films from the States exerts a compulsive force.

fearfully—both insomniacs, both heat intolerant, both restless night readers—and wondered how we would survive
the long nights, unable even to distract ourselves by reading.

I tossed and turned all night, kept awake in part by the
heat and humidity; in part by a strange visual excitement
such as I am sometimes prone to, especially at the start of a
migraine—endlessly moving vistas of breadfruit trees and
bananas on the darkened ceiling; and, not least, by a sense
of intoxication and delight that now, finally, I had arrived
on the island of the colorblind.

None of us slept well that night. We gathered, tousled,
on the terrace at dawn, and decided to reconnoiter a bit. I
took my notebook and made brief notes as we walked
(though the ink tended to smudge in the wet air):

Six o'clock in the morning, and though the air is blood-
hot, sapping, doldrum-still, the island is already alive with
activity—pigs squealing, scampering through the undergrowth; smells of fish and taro cooking; repairing the roofs
of houses with palm fronds and banana leaves as Pingelap
prepares itself for a new day. Three men are working on a
canoe—a lovely traditional shape, sawn and shaved from a
single massive tree trunk, using materials and methods
which have not changed in a thousand or more years. Bob
and Knut are fascinated by the boat building, and watch it
closely, contentedly. Knut's attention is also drawn to the
other side of the road, to the graves and altars beside some
of the houses. There is no communal burial, no graveyard,

in Pingelap, only this cozy burying of the dead next to their houses, so that they still remain, almost palpably, part of the family. There are strings, like clotheslines, hung around the graves, upon which gaily colored and patterned pieces of cloth have been hung—perhaps to keep demons away, perhaps just for decoration; I am not sure, but they seem festive in spirit.

My own attention is riveted by the enormous density of vegetation all around us, so much denser than any temperate forest, and a brilliant yellow lichen on some of the trees. I nibble at it—many lichens are edible- –but it is bitter and unpromising.

Everywhere we saw breadfruit trees—sometimes whole groves of them, with their large, deeply lobed leaves; they were heavy with the giant fruits which Dampier, three hundred years ago, had likened to loaves of bread. I had never seen trees so generous of themselves—they were very easy to grow, James had said, and each tree might yield a hundred massive fruits a year, more than enough to sustain a man. A single tree would bear fruit for fifty years or more, and then its fine wood could be used for lumber, especially for building the hulls of canoes.

Down by the reef, dozens of children were already swimming, some of them toddlers, barely able to walk, but plunging fearlessly into the water, among the sharp corals, shouting with excitement. I saw two or three achromatopic kids diving and romping and yelling with the rest—they did not seem isolated or set apart, at least at this

stage of their lives, and since it was still very early, and the
sky was overcast, they were not blinded as they would be
later in the day. Some of the larger children had tied the
rubber soles of old sandals to their hands, and had developed a remarkably swift dog paddle using these. Others
dived to the bottom, which was thick with huge, tumid sea
cucumbers, and used these to squeeze jets of water at each
other. . . . I am fond of holothurians, and I hoped they
would survive.

I waded into the water, and started diving for sea
cucumbers myself. At one time, I had read, there had been
a brisk trade exporting sea cucumbers to Malaya, China,
and Japan, where they are highly esteemed as trepang or
bêche-de-mer or namako. I myself love a good sea cucum-
ber on occasion—they have a tough gelatinousness, an animal cellulose in their tissues, which I find most appealing.
Carrying one back to the beach, I asked James whether the
Pingelapese ate them much. "We eat them," he said, "but
they are tough and need a lot of cooking—though this
one," he pointed to the *Stichopus* I had dredged up, "you
can eat raw." I sank my teeth into it, wonder if he was joking; I found it impossible to get through the leathery
integument—it was like trying to eat an old, weathered
shoe.[5]

[5]Many holothurians have very sharp, microscopic spicules in their body walls;
these spicules take all sorts of shapes—one sees button granules, ellipsoids,
bars, racquets, wheel forms with spokes, and anchors. If the spicules (especially
the anchor-shaped ones, which are as perfect and sharp as any boat anchor) are

After breakfast, we visited a local family, the Edwards. Entis Edward is achromatopic, as are all three of his children, from a babe in arms, who was squinting in the bright sunlight, to a girl of eleven. His wife, Emma, has normal vision, though she evidently is a carrier of the gene. Entis is well educated, with little command of English but a natural eloquence; he is a minister in the Congregationalist Church and a fisherman, a man well respected in the community. But this, his wife told us, was far from the rule. Most of those born with the maskun never learn to read, because they cannot see the teacher's writing on the board; they have less chance of marrying—partly because it is recognized that their children are likelier to be affected, partly because they cannot work outdoors in the bright sunlight, as most of the islanders do.[6] Entis was an exception here,

---

not dissolved or destroyed (many hours, or even days, of boiling may be needed), they may lodge in the gut lining of the unfortunate eater, causing serious but invisible bleeding. This has been used to murderous effect for many centuries in China, where trepang is regarded as a great delicacy.

[6]Irene Maumenee Hussels and her colleagues at Johns Hopkins have taken samples of blood from the entire population of Pingelap and from many Pingelapese in Pohnpei and Mokil. Using DNA analysis, they hope it will be possible to locate the genetic abnormality which causes the maskun. If this is achieved, it will then be possible to identify carriers of the disease—but this, Maumenee Hussels points out, will raise complex ethical and cultural questions. It may be, for example, that such identification would militate against chances of marriage or employment for the thirty percent of the population that carries the gene.

on every count, and very conscious of it: "I have been lucky," he said. "It is not easy for the others."

Apart from the social problems it causes, Entis does not feel his colorblindness a disability, though he is often disabled by his intolerance of bright light and his inability to see fine detail. Knut nodded as he heard this; he had been deeply attentive to everything Entis said, and identified with him in many ways. He took out his monocular to show Entis—the monocular which is almost like a third eye for him, and always hangs round his neck. Entis's face lit up with delight as, adjusting the focus, he could see, for the first time, boats bobbing on the water, trees on the horizon, the faces of people on the other side of the road, and, focusing right down, the details of the skin whorls on his own fingertips. Impulsively, Knut removed the monocular from around his neck, and presented it to Entis. Entis, clearly moved, said nothing, but his wife went into the house and came out bearing a beautiful necklace she had made, a triple chain of matched cowrie shells, the most precious thing the family had, and this she solemnly presented to Knut, while Entis looked on.

Knut himself was now disabled, without his monocular—"It is like giving half my eye to him, because it is necessary to my vision"—but deeply happy. "It will make all the difference to him," he said. "I'll get another one later."

The following day we saw James, squinting against the sunlight, watching a group of teenagers playing basketball. As our interpreter and guide, he had seemed cheerful, sociable, knowledgeable, very much part of the community—but now, for the first time, he seemed quiet, wistful, and rather solitary and sad. We got to talking, and more of his story emerged. Life and school had been difficult for him, as for the other achromatopes on Pingelap—unshielded sunlight was literally blinding for him, and he could hardly go out into it without a dark cloth over his eyes. He could not join the rough-and-tumble, the open-air games the other children enjoyed. His acuity was very poor, and he could not see any of the schoolbooks unless he held them three inches from his eyes. Nonetheless he was exceptionally intelligent and resourceful, and he learned to read early, and loved reading, despite this handicap. Like Delihda, he had gone to Pohnpei for further schooling (Pingelap itself has a small elementary school, but not secondary education). Clever, ambitious, aspiring to a larger life, James went on to get a scholarship to the University of Guam, spent five years there, and got a degree in sociology. He had returned to Pingelap full of brave ideas: to help the islanders market their wares more efficiently, to obtain better medical services and child care, to bring electricity and running water into every house, to improve standards of education, to bring a new political consciousness and pride to the island, and to make sure that every islander—the achromatopes especially—would get as a birthright the literacy and education he had had to struggle so hard to achieve.

None of this had panned out—he encountered an enormous inertia and resistance to change, a lack of ambition, a laissez-faire, and gradually he himself had ceased to strive. He could find no job on Pingelap appropriate to his education or talents, because Pingelap, with its subsistence economy, *has* no jobs, apart from those of the health worker, the magistrate, and a couple of teachers. And now, with his university accent, his new manners and outlook, James no longer completely belonged to the small world he had left, and found himself set apart, an outsider.

We had seen a beautifully patterned mat outside the Edwards' house, and now noticed similar ones everywhere, in front of the traditional thatched houses, and equally the newer ones, made of concrete blocks with corrugated aluminum roofs. The weaving of these mats was a craft unchanged from "the time before time," James told us; the traditional fibers, made from palm fronds, were still used (although the traditional vegetable dyes had been replaced by an inky blue obtained from surplus carbon paper, for which the islanders otherwise had little need). The island's finest weaver was a colorblind woman, who had learned the craft from her mother, who was also colorblind. James took us to meet her; she was doing her intricate work inside a hut so dark we could hardly see anything after the bright sunlight. (Knut, on the othe hand, took off his double sunglasses and said it was, visually, the most comfortable place he had yet encountered on the island.) As we adapted to the darkness, we began to see her special art of brightnesses, delicate patterns of differing luminances, patterns that all but disappeared as soon as we took one of her mats into the sunlight outside.

Recently, Knut told her, his sister, Britt, to prove it could be done, had knitted a jacket in sixteen different colors. She had devised her own system for keeping track of the skeins of wool, by labeling them with numbers. The jacket had marvelous intricate patterns and images drawn from Norwegian folktales, he said, but since they were done in dim browns and purples, colors without much chromatic contrast, they were almost invisible to normal eyes. Britt, however, responding to luminances only, could see them quite clearly, perhaps even more clearly than color-normals. "It is my special, secret art," she says. "You have to be totally colorblind to see it."

Later in the day, we went to the island's dispensary to meet more people with the maskun—almost forty people were there, more than half the achromatopes on the island. We set up in the main room—Bob with his ophthalmoscope, his lenses and acuity tests, and I with a mass of colored yarns and drawings and pens, as well as the standard color-testing kits. Knut had brought along a set of Sloan achromatopsia cards. I had never seen these before, and Knut explained the test to me: "Each of these cards has a range of grey squares which vary only in tone, progressing from a very light grey to a very dark grey, almost black, really. Each square has a hole cut out in the center, and if I place a sheet of colored paper behind these—like this—one of the squares will be a match for the color; they will have an equal density." He pointed to an orange dot, surrounded by a medium grey background. "For me the internal dot and the surround here are exactly the same."

Such a match would be completely meaningless for a color-normal, for whom no color can ever "match" a grey, and extremely difficult for most—but quite easy and natural for an achromatope, who sees all colors, and all greys, only as differing luminances. Ideally, the test should be administered with a standard source of illumination, but since there was no electricity to run lights on the island, Knut had to use himself as a standard, comparing each achromatope's responses to his own. In nearly every case, these were the same, or very close.

Medical testing is usually rather private, but here it was very public, and with dozens of youngsters peering in through the windows, or wandering among us as we tested, took on a communal and humorous and almost festive quality.

Bob wanted to check refraction in each person, and to examine their retinas closely—by no means easy, when the eyes are continually jerking with nystagmus. It was not possible, of course, to see the microscopic rods and cones (or lack thereof) directly, but he could find nothing else amiss on inspection with his ophthalmoscope. It had been suggested by some earlier researchers that the maskun was linked with severe myopia; but Bob found that although many of the achromatopes were nearsighted, many were not (Knut himself is rather farsighted)—and he also found that a similar proportion of the island's color-normals were nearsighted as well. If there were a genetic form of myopia here, Bob felt, it was transmitted independently of the achromatopsia.[7] It was possible as well, he added, that reports of nearsightedness had been exaggerated by earlier researchers who had observed so many of the islanders squinting and bringing small objects closer to view— behaviors which might appear to indicate myopia but actually reflected the intolerance of bright light and poor acuity of the achromatopes.

I asked the achromatopes if they could judge the colors of various yarns, or at least match them with one another. The matching was clearly done on the basis of brightness and not color—thus yellow and pale blue might be grouped with white, or saturated reds and greens with black. I had also brought the Ishihara pseudoisochromatic test plates for ordinary partial colorblindness, which have numbers and

---

[7]In 1970 Maumenee Hussels and Morton came to Pingelap with a team of geneticists from the University of Hawaii. They came on the MS *Microglory*, bringing sophisticated equipment, including an electroretinogram for measuring the retina's response to flashes of light. The retinas of those with the maskun, they found, showed normal responses from the rods, but no response whatsoever from the cones—but it was not until 1994 that Donald Miller and David Williams at the University of Rochester described the first direct observation of retinal cones in living subjects. Since then, they have used techniques from astronomy, adaptive optics, to allow routine imaging of the moving eye. This equipment has not yet been used to examine any congenital achromatopes, but it would be interesting to do so, to see whether the absence or defect of cones can be visualized directly.

Intriguingly, as Gustavo Aguirre and his colleagues at Cornell University have been investigating, there is a strain of Alaskan malamute dogs who exhibit severe day-blindness (hemeralopia) by the age of eight to ten weeks; in these

figures formed by colored dots, distinguishable only by color (and not luminosity) from the dots surrounding them. Some of the Ishihara plates, paradoxically, cannot be seen by color-normals, but only by achromatopes—these have dots which are identical in hue, but vary slightly in luminance. The older children with the maskun were particularly excited by these—it turned the tables on me, the tester—and they jostled to take their turns pointing out the special numbers that I could not see.

Knut's presence while we were examining those with maskun, his sharing of his own experiences, was crucial, for it helped remove our questions from the sphere of the inquisitive, the impersonal, and bring us all together as fellow creatures, making it easier for us, finally, to clarify and reassure. For although the lack of color vision in itself did not seem to be a subject of concern, there were many misapprehensions about the maskun—in particular, fears that the disease might be progressive, might lead to complete blindness, might go along with retardation, madness, epilepsy, or heart trouble. Some believed that it could be

dogs the retinal cones degenerate early and disappear. Like human beings with maskun, such dogs show day-blindness and total colorblindness, but—unlike achromatopes—do not have a profound loss of visual acuity, because canines lack a foveomacular region in the retina and thus do not encounter problems with foveal fixation. Like human maskun, this canine hemeralopia is inherited as an autosomal recessive, and preliminary work seems to pinpoint a specific gene in the disease process. "It will be interesting," Aguirre notes, "once we identify the gene and the mutation in the dog, to establish whether or not the Pingelap islanders and other human achromatopes have a mutation in the same gene."

caused by carelessness during pregnancy, or transmitted through a sort of contagion. Though there was some sense of the fact that the maskun tended to run in certain families, there was little or no knowledge about recessive genes and heredity. Bob and I did our best to stress that the maskun was nonprogressive, affected only certain aspects of vision, and that with a few simple optical aids—dark sunglasses or visors to reduce bright light, and magnifying glasses and monoculars to allow reading and sharp distance vision—someone with the maskun could go through school, live, travel, work, in much the same way as anyone else. But more than words could, Knut himself brought this home, partly by using his own sunglasses and magnifier, partly by the manifest achievement and freedom of his own life.

Outside the dispensary, we began to give out the wraparound sunglasses we had brought, along with hats and visors, with varying results. One mother, with an achromatopic infant squalling and blinking in her arms, took a pair of tiny sunglasses and put them on the baby's nose, which seemed to calm him, and led to an immediate change in his behavior. No longer blinking and squinting, he opened his eyes wide and began to gaze around with a lively curiosity. One old woman, the oldest achromatope on the island, indignantly refused to try any sunglasses on. She had lived eighty years as she was, she said, and was not about to start wearing sunglasses now. But many of the other achromatopic adults and teenagers evidently liked the sunglasses, wrinkling their noses at the unaccustomed weight of them, but manifested less disabled by the bright light.

It is said that Wittgenstein was either the easiest or the most difficult of houseguests to accommodate, because though he would eat, with gusto, whatever was served to him on his arrival, he would then want exactly the same for every subsequent meal for the rest of his stay. This is seen as extraordinary, even pathological, by many people— but since I myself am similarly disposed, I see it as perfectly normal. Indeed, having a sort of passion for monotony, I greatly enjoyed the unvarying meals on Pingelap, whereas Knut and Bob longed for variety. Our first meal, the model which was to be repeated three times daily, consisted of taro, bananas, pandanus, breadfruit, yams, and tuna followed by papaya and young coconuts full of milk. Since I am a fish and banana person anyhow, these meals were wholly to my taste.

But we were all revolted by the Spam which appeared with each meal—invariably fried; why, I wondered, should the Pingelapese eat this filthy stuff when their own basic diet was both healthy and delicious? Especially when they could hardly afford it, because Pingelap has only the small amount of money it can raise from the export of copra, mats, and pandanus fruits to Pohnpei. I had talked with the unctuous Spam baron on the plane; and now, on Pingelap, I could see the addiction in full force. How was it that not only the Pingelapese, but all the peoples of the Pacific, seemingly, could fall so helplessly, so voraciously, on this stuff, despite its intolerable cost to their budgets and their health? I was not the first to puzzle about this; later, when I came to read Paul Theroux's book *The Happy Isles of Oceania*, I found his hypothesis about this universal Spam mania:

> It was a theory of mine that former cannibals of Oceania now feasted on Spam because Spam came the nearest to approximating the porky taste of human flesh. "Long pig" as they called a cooked human being in much of Melanesia. It was a fact that the people-eaters of the Pacific had all evolved, or perhaps degenerated, into Spam-eaters. And in the absense of Spam they settled for corned beef, which also had a corpsy flavor.

> So far as I knew, though, there was no tradition of cannibalism on Pingelap.

Whether or not Spam is, as Theroux suggests, a sublimate of cannibalism, it was a relief to visit the taro patch, the ultimate source of food, which covers ten swampy acres in the center of the island. The Pingelapese speak of taro with reverence and affection, and sooner or later everyone takes a turn at working in the communally owned patch. The ground is carefully cleaned of debris, and turned over by hand, and the soil is then planted with shoots about eighteen inches long. The plants grow with extraordinary speed, soon reaching ten feet or more in height, with broad triangular leaves arching overhead. The upkeep of the patch devolves traditionally on the women, working barefoot in the ankle-high mud, and different parts of the patch are tended and harvested by them each day. The deep shade cast by the huge leaves makes it a favorite meeting place, particularly for those with the maskun.

A dozen or more varieties of taro are grown in the patch, and their large, starchy roots range in taste from bitter to sweet. The roots can be eaten fresh, or dried and stored for later use. Taro is the ultimate crop for Pingelap, and there is still a vivid communal memory of how, during typhoon Lengkieki two centuries ago, the taro patch was inundated with salt water and totally destroyed—and that it was this which brought the remaining islanders to starvation.

Coming back from the taro patch, we were approached by an old man in the woods, who came up to us diffidently, but determinedly, and asked if he could get Bob's advice, as he was going blind. He had clouded eyes, and Bob, examining him later at the dispensary with his ophthalmoscope, confirmed that he had cataracts, but could find nothing else amiss. Surgery could probably help him, he told the old man, and this could be done in the hospital on Pohnpei, with every chance of restoring good vision. The old man gave us a big smile and hugged Bob. When Bob asked Delihda, who coordinates with the visiting nurse from Pohnpei, to put the man's name down for cataract surgery, she commented that it was a good thing he had approached us. If he had not, she said, he would have been allowed to go completely blind. Medical services in Pingelap are spread very thin, already overstretched by more pressing conditions. Cataracts (like achromatopsia) are a very low-priority concern here; and cataract surgery, with the added costs of transport to Pohnpei, is generally considered too expensive to do. So the old man would get treatment, but he would be the exception to the rule.

I counted five churches on Pingelap, all Congregationalist. I had not seen so great a density of churches since being in the little Mennonite community of La Crete in Alberta; here, as there, churchgoing is universal. And when there is not churchgoing, there is hymn singing and Sunday school.

The spiritual invasion of the island began in earnest in the mid-nineteenth century, and by 1880, the entire population had been converted. But even now, more than five generations later, though Christianity is incorporated into the culture, and fervently embraced in a sense, there is still a reverence and nostalgia for the old ways, rooted in the soil and vegetation, the history and geography, of the island. Wandering through the dense forest at one point, we heard voices singing—voices so high and unexpected and unearthly and pure that I again had a sense of Pingelap as a place of enchantment, another world, an island of spirits. Making our way through the thick undergrowth, we reached a little clearing, where a dozen children stood with their teacher, singing hymns in the morning sun. Or were they singing *to* the morning sun? The words were Christian, but the setting, the feeling, were mythical and pagan. We kept hearing snatches of song as we walked about the island, usually without seeing the singer or singers—choirs, voices, incorporeal, on the air. They seemed innocent at first, almost angelic, but then to take on an ambiguous, mocking note. If I had thought first of Ariel, I thought now of Caliban; and whenever voices, hallucination-like, filled the air, Pingelap, for me, took on the quality of Prospero's isle:

> Be not afeared: the isle is full of noises,
> Sounds and sweet airs, that give delight, and hurt not.

When Jane Hurd, an anthropologist, spent two years among the Pingelapese on Pohnpei in 1968 and '69, the old nahnmwarki was still able to give her, in the form of an extended epic poem, an entire oral history of the island—but with his death a good deal of this knowledge and memory died. The present nahnmwarki can give the flavor of old Pingelapese belief and myth, but no longer has the detailed knowledge his grandfather had. Nonetheless, he himself, as a teacher at the school, does his best to give the children a sense of their heritage and of the pre-Christian culture which once flourished on the island. He spoke nostalgically, it seemed to us, of the old days on Pingelap, when everyone knew who they were, where they came from, and how the island came into being. At one time, the myth went, the three islets of Pingelap formed a single piece of land, with its own god, Isopaw. When an alien god came from a distant island and split Pingelap into two, Isopaw chased him away—and the third islet was created from a handful of sand dropped in the chase.

We were struck by the multiple systems of belief, some seemingly contradictory, which coexist among the Pingelapese. A mythical history of the island is maintained alongside its secular history; thus the maskun is seen simultaneously in mystical terms (as a curse visited upon the sinful or disobedient) and in purely biological terms (as a morally neutral, genetic condition transmitted from generation to generation). Traditionally, it was traced back to the Nahnmwarki Okonomwaun, who ruled from 1822 to 1870, and his wife, Dokas. Of their six children, two were achromatopic. The myth explaining this was recorded by Irene Maumenee Hussels and Newton Morton, geneticists from the University of Hawaii who visited Pingelap (and worked with Hurd) in the late 1960s:

> The god Isoahpahu became enamored of Dokas and instructed Okonomwaun to appropriate her. From time to time, Isoahpahu appeared in the guise of Okonomwaun and had intercourse with Dokas, fathering the affected children, while the normal children came from Okonomwaun. Isoahpahu loved other Pingelapese women and had

affected children by them. The "proof" of this is that persons with achromatopsia shun the light but have relatively good night vision, like their ghostly ancestor.

There were other indigenous myths about the maskun: that it might arise if a pregnant woman walked upon the beach in the middle of the day—the blazing sun, it was felt, might partly blind the unborn child in the womb. Yet another legend had it that it came from a descendant of the Nahnmwarki Mwahuele, who had survived typhoon Lengkieki. This descendant, Inek, was trained as a Christian minister by a missionary, Mr. Doane, and was assigned to Chuuk, as Hussels and Morton write, but refused to move because of his large family on Pingelap. Mr. Doane, "angered by this lack of evangelical zeal," cursed Inek and his children with the maskun.

There were also persistent notions, as always with disease, that the maskun had come from the outside world. The nahnmwarki spoke, in this vein, of how a number of Pingelapese had been forced to labor in the German phosphate mines on the distant island of Nauru, and then, on their return, had fathered children with maskun. The myth of contamination, ascribed (like so many other ills) to the coming of the white man, took on a new form with our visit. This was the first time the Pingelapese had ever seen another achromatope, an achromatope from outside, and this "confirmed" their brooding suspicions. Two days after our arrival, a revised myth had already taken root in the Pingelapese lore: it must have been achromatopic white whalers from the far north, they now realized, who had landed on Pingelap early in the last century—raping and rampaging among the island women, fathering dozens of achromatopic children, and bringing their white man's curse to the island. The Pingelapese with maskun, by this reckoning, were partly Norwegian—descendants of people like Knut. Knut was awed by the rapidity with which this not entirely jocular, fantastic myth emerged, and by finding himself, or his people, "revealed" as the ultimate origin of the maskun.

On our last evening in Pingelap, a huge crimson sunset shot with purples and yellows and a touch of green hung over the ocean and filled half the sky. Even Knut exclaimed, "Unbelievable!" and said he had never seen such a sunset before. As we came down to the shore, we saw dozens of people almost submerged in the water—only their heads were visible above the reef. This happened every evening, James had told us—it was the only way to cool off. Looking around, we saw others lying, sitting, standing and chatting in small clusters—it looked as if most of the island's population was here. The cooling hour, the social hour, the hour of immersion, had begun.

As it got darker, Knut and the achromatopic islanders moved more easily. It is common knowledge among the Pingelapese that those with the maskun manage better at scotopic times—dusk and dawn, and moonlit nights—and for this reason, they are often employed as night fishers.

And in this the achromatopes are preeminent; they seem able to see the fish in their dim course underwater, the glint of moonlight on their outstretched fins as they leap—as well as, or perhaps better than, anyone else.

Our last night was an ideal one for the night fishers. I had hoped we might go in one of the enormous hollow-log canoes with outriggers which we had seen earlier, but we were led instead toward a boat with a small outboard motor. The air was very warm and still, so it was sweet to feel a slight breeze as we moved out. As we glided into deeper waters, the shoreline of Pingelap vanished from sight, and we moved on a vast lightless swell with only the stars and the great arc of the Milky Way overhead.

Our helmsman knew all the major stars and constellations, seemed completely at home with the heavens—Knut, indeed, was the only one equally knowledgeable, and the two of them exchanged their knowledge in whispers: Knut with all modern astronomy at his fingertips, the helmsman with an ancient practical knowledge such as had enabled the Micronesians and Polynesians, a thousand years ago, to sail across the immensities of the Pacific by celestial navigation alone, in voyages comparable to interplanetary travel, until, at last, they discovered islands, homes, as rare and far apart as planets in the cosmos.

About eight o'clock the moon rose, almost full, and so brilliant that it seemed to eclipse the stars. We heard the splash of flying fish as they arced out of the water, dozens at a time, and the plopping sound as they plummeted back to the surface.

The waters of the Pacific are full of a tiny protozoan, *Noctiluca*, a bioluminescent creature able to generate light, like a firefly. It was Knut who first noticed their phosphorescence in the water—a phosphorescence most evident when the water was disturbed. Sometimes when the flying fish leapt out of the water, they would leave a luminous disturbance, a glowing wake, as they did so—and another splash of light as they landed.[8]

Night fishing used to be done with a flaming torch; now it is done with the help of a flashlight, the light serving to dazzle as well as spot the fish. As the beautiful creatures were illuminated in a blinding flashlight beam, I was reminded how, as a child, I would see German planes transfixed by roving searchlights as they flew in the darkened skies over London. One by one we pursued the fish; we followed their careerings relentlessly, this way and that, until we

---

[8]There may be as many as thirty thousand of these tiny bioluminescent creatures in a cubic foot of seawater, and many observers have attested to the extraordinary brilliance of seas filled with *Noctiluca*. Charles Frederick Holder, in his 1887 *Living Lights: A Popular Account of Phosphorescent Animals and Vegetables*, relates how M. de Tessan described the phosphorescent waves as "appearing like the vivid flashes of lightning," giving enough illumination to read by:

> It lighted up the chamber that I and my companions occupied [de Tessan wrote] . . . though it was situated more than fifty yards distant from the breakers. I even attempted to write by the light, but the flashes were of too short duration.

Holder continues his account of these "living asteroids":

> When a vessel is ploughing through masses of these animals, the effect is extremely brilliant. An American captain states that when his ship traversed a zone of these animals in the Indian Ocean, nearly thirty miles in extent, the light emitted by these myriads of fire-bodies . . . eclipsed the brightest stars; the milky way was but dimly seen; and as far

could draw close enough for the fisher to shoot out the great hoop of his net, and catch them as they returned to the water. They accumulated in the bottom of the boat, silvery, squirming, until they were hit on the head (though one, actually, in its frenzy, managed to leap out of the boat, and we so admired this that we did not try to catch it again).

After an hour we had enough, and it was time to go after deeper-water fish. There were two teenage boys with us, one achromatopic, and they now donned scuba gear and masks and, clutching spears and flashlights, went over the side of the boat. We could see them, two hundred yards or more from the boat, like luminous fish, the phosphorescent waters outlining their bodies as they moved. After ten minutes they returned, loaded with the fish they had speared, and climbed back into the boat, their wet scuba gear gleaming blackly in the moonlight.

---

as the eye could reach the water presented the appearance of a vast, gleaming sea of molten metal, of purest white. The sails, masts, and rigging cast weird shadows all about; flames sprang from the bow as the ship surged along, and great waves of living light spread out ahead—a fascinating and appalling sight. . . .

The light of Noctilucae in full vigor is a clear blue; but, if the water is agitated, it becames nearly, if not quite white, producing rich silvery gleams sprinkled with greenish and bluish spangles.

Humboldt also describes this phenomenon, in his *Views of Nature:*

In the ocean, gelatinous sea-worms, living and dead, shine like luminous stars, converting by their phosphorescent light the green surface of the ocean into one vast sheet of fire. Indelible is the impression left on my mind by those calm tropical nights in the Pacific, where the constellation of Argo in its zenith, and the setting Southern Cross, pour their mild planetary light through the ethereal azure of the sky, while dolphins mark the foaming waves with their luminous furrows.

The long, slow trip back was very peaceful—we lay back in the boat; the fishers murmured softly among themselves. We had enough, more than enough, fish for all. Fires would be lit on the long sandy beach, and we would have a grand, final feast on Pingelap before flying back to Pohnpei the next morning. We reached the shore and waded back onto the beach, pulling the boat up behind us. The sand itself, broader with the tide's retreat, was still wet with the phosphorescent sea, and now, as we walked upon it, our footsteps left a luminous spoor.

# VINTAGE BOOKS BY OLIVER SACKS

*An Anthropologist on Mars*

In these seven paradoxical tales of neurological disorder and creativity, Sacks transports us into the uncanny worlds of his subjects, including an artist who loses his ability to see (or even imagine) color, and a surgeon who performs delicate operations in spite of the compulsive tics and outbursts of his Tourette's syndrome.

Psychology/Literature/0-679-75697-3

*Awakenings*

In the spring of 1969, Oliver Sacks initiated L-DOPA drug treatment for the post-encephalitic residents of Mount Carmel hospital, many of whom had been "frozen" and catatonic for decades. The drug had an astonishing, explosive, "awakening" effect, but the challenges of awakening to a changed world raised profound questions about medical care and what gives meaning to a life.

Psychology/Literature/0-375-70405-1

*The Island of the Colorblind*

Part travelogue, part medical mystery story, this is an account in which Sacks's journeys to a tiny Pacific atoll and the island of Guam become explorations of the meaning of islands, the genesis of disease, the wonders of botany, the nature of deep geological time, and the complexities of being human.

Science/Literature/0-375-70073-0

## Migraine

*Migraine* is Sacks's classic meditation on the nature of health and malady, on the unity of mind and body. Here too is Sacks's discovery of how migraine may show us, through hallucinatory displays, the elemental activity of the cerebral cortex—and, potentially, the self-organizing patterns of Nature itself.

Psychology/Literature/0-375-70406-X

## Seeing Voices

In *Seeing Voices* Oliver Sacks turns his attention to the subject of deafness, and the result is a deeply felt portrait of a minority struggling for recognition and respect—a minority with its own rich, sometimes astonishing culture and its own unique visual language, an extraordinary mode of communication that tells us much about the basis of language in hearing people as well.

Psychology/Literature/0-375-70407-8

## Uncle Tungsten: Memories of a Chemical Boyhood

Oliver Sacks's memoir of his childhood in London in the 1930s and '40s, this is the story of a brilliant young mind springing to life. By turns elegiac and comic, *Uncle Tungsten* chronicles Sacks's love affair with science and the magnificently odd and sometimes harrowing childhood in which that love affair unfolded.

Science/Memoir/0-375-70404-3